# The Pharmacist Is IN; Answers to Health Questions You Didn't Know You Had

Jeannie Collins Beaudin

Published by Collins Pharmacy Ltd., 2021.

THE PHARMACIST IS IN; ANSWERS TO HEALTH QUESTIONS YOU DIDN'T KNOW YOU HAD

**First edition. May 7, 2021.**



ISBN: 979-8201553579

Written by Jeannie Collins Beaudin.

# Table of Contents


Introduction.................................................................................................1

Chapter 1: What can I do to Improve My Lifestyle and Enjoy Life More?.......3

Chapter 2: What if I Have Stomach Problems?..................................... 19

Chapter 3: Are Herbal (Natural) Medications Safe to Take? ............................ 23

Chapter 4: How Can I Prevent Heart Disease and Stroke? ............................... 27

Chapter 5: Are Microbes in Our Gut Important?....................................... 39

Chapter 6: What Does Vitamin K2 Do?  Is It Important For Our Health?... 47

Chapter 7: Is it Dangerous to Be Overweight? ...................................... 51

Chapter 8: The Environment: Where do Drugs We Swallow Eventually Go?.................................................................................................. 55

Chapter 9: What Activities Can Help Us Live Healthier and Longer?........... 67

Chapter 10: How Can I Improve My Memory? .................................... 75

Chapter 11: How Can I Reduce My Risk of Stress, Anxiety and Depression? .............................................................................................. 87

Chapter 12: The Last Word..................................................... 99

This book is dedicated to all the faithful readers of my weekly blog.
You make it all worthwhile!

Cover design by Michelle Beaudin

# Introduction

Many of us take our health for granted. Sometimes it's a milestone birthday or a health crisis that starts us thinking about what we can do to stay healthy or to regain our health and fitness. If you're reading this, perhaps you're in one of those places.

For me, it was turning 40 but, as I had just opened my pharmacy, it wasn't much more than thinking and reading about it. As menopause loomed, hormones became an area of interest for me and I started reading books and taking courses on the subject. I began sharing what I had learned — becoming a specialty pharmacist, helping clients make their transition through the "Change" easier. But personally, I had made no substantial changes. I was simply in "questioning mode"... What should I be doing to make sure I don't have a miserable menopause?

But when my husband was 50, he had a heart attack. That health crisis that made both of us want to get serious about improving our health and our lifestyle. While he was still in the hospital, I gave him a little gift — a cookbook from the American Heart Association. Its first section is all about making choices that will lower heart disease risk. We quickly changed our diet when he came home, eliminating trans fats and reducing salt. We started exercising more and worked on reducing our stress levels.

When I look back, stress was probably the most important factor in my husband's development of heart disease, as we juggled family and work responsibilities. We have three children, and my husband was teaching full time plus managing two pharmacies. Then he started an accounting course - all at the same time! The stress of not being able to keep up became overwhelming, leading to a heart attack.

Now, 15 years later, we are retired and gradually simplifying our lives... enjoying retirement and some travelling. Stress can still creep in, but we talk through it together to keep everything in perspective. Experts tell us: it isn't the stress itself, it's your reaction to the stress that can damage your health.

We see our doctors at least once a year to monitor our health, and to catch and treat any negative change as soon as possible. My husband likes to say: you take your car in for a yearly inspection, get regular tune ups and investigate anything unusual right away before it becomes a big problem — and you need to do the same for your body!

So, now you know me a little—the lifestyle I'm trying to shape, what my goals are and a bit of where I'm coming from. I'd like this to be a "chat" with you, somewhat like I've had with so many clients I knew well, hanging out at the pharmacy counter for a while, visiting with me when it wasn't busy.

The following chapters are answers to some questions I've had about staying healthy and my pharmacy clients were interested in these kinds of questions, too. I'm sure you have similar questions, although you may not have taken time to consider them or research the answers.

Some chapters are about new health discoveries or controversies that surprised me as a pharmacist. Science constantly changes as we learn more. And sometimes, like the "surprise" pandemic, scientists have been warning of the potential for problems for years... if we'd only listen.

We all want to continue to feel young and energetic, enjoying life well into old age. I hope you find answers and interesting ideas you can use in these pages. I've also included thoughts on keeping the planet healthy - we can't have optimum health if we live in a contaminated environment. And I've included links to the information sources I used while writing, so you can read further on topics that interest you...

As with any health information you read, never change your treatment without discussing it with your doctor first. He or she is the ideal person to help you customize your health plan, according to your individual characteristics, and ensure you are making the best choices for your health.

# Chapter 1: What can I do to Improve My Lifestyle and Enjoy Life More?

## Exercise

*"If it was a pill, exercise would be a trillion-dollar money-maker prescribed to everyone."*

— Dr. Scott Lear, heart disease prevention researcher at Simon Fraser University, British Columbia, Canada.

Exercise is so effective at preventing and improving some chronic illnesses, doctors are being encouraged to write prescriptions for it. Exercise decreases the risk of many diseases, including heart disease, stroke, Type 2 diabetes, depression[1], and many cancers. Moving Medicine[2] is a beta site being developed to encourage doctors to "prescribe" exercise to their patients. Here are a few statistics showing how much exercise can lower chronic disease risk, as quoted on their website:

- Type 2 diabetes - decreases risk by 40%

- Cardiovascular disease - decreases risk by 35%

- Falls -30% less risk of falling

- Dementia - decreases risk by 30%

- Depression - 30% less risk of low mood

- Joint and back pain - decreases occurrence by 20%

Physical activity is as important for health as many medications, but without the side effects. Humans were made to move, and experts believe inactivity to be as harmful to our health as cigarettes. But the more affluent our society becomes, the less most of us move.

A global study of activity found that, on average, over one-quarter of adults worldwide are not getting enough physical activity. And high-income Western countries (like us in North America) have inactivity rates twice as high as those of poorer countries. Over 50% of people in some areas of North America are not active enough for optimum health.

And women are less active than men on average—up to 20% less in some countries. A 2017 survey published in Health Reports[3] found that only 2% of girls aged 12-17 met the Canadian Movement Guidelines that include adequate sleep and at least 60 minutes of moderate to vigorous activity. A Dalhousie University study noted that teenage girls worry about appearances when they exercise: they want to be pretty but natural-looking, thin but not too skinny, fit but not too muscular. Their responses in the study suggest that outdoor activities can provide an important venue to feel comfortable, safe and confident doing physical activity, compared to a gym setting where, as self-conscious teenagers, they felt they needed to worry more about clothing and appearances.

There is statistical evidence that inactivity is worsening in too many areas year by year. With a corresponding increase in chronic diseases like diabetes and heart disease, it is time to create strategies to increase physical activity levels across populations and on a personal level.

Community infrastructure can influence activity in the young and old. Open spaces, like parks and walking/biking paths, provide enjoyable and convenient opportunities for physical activity. A visible example is the throngs of people who use the skating oval added to the park known as the Commons in downtown Halifax, Nova Scotia, Canada. You can even borrow skates and helmets there for free! This facility is an excellent model that other cities should adopt to improve the health of its citizens. Public bike rentals are another model popular in some countries, where bikes are available for pickup and drop-off at various locations to enable use as transportation or for leisure activity.

High quality public transport and incentives to use it, rather than motorized vehicles, can produce an overall increase in daily activity of a population. I noticed a marked increase in my activity level when using public transit while travelling in Europe, just by walking to and from the nearest system access.

So, if you want to reduce your chances of developing a chronic disease as you age, look for ways to add more exercise into your day — and it doesn't have to be a session at the gym. Remember that experts say ten minutes of activity three times a day is equal to a single 30-minute session. Park farther away from the door when doing errands or take the stairs instead of the elevator—it all adds up. My husband and I enjoy a daily 30-minute walk to check our mailbox most days, and climbing up and down the stairs in our 3-story house adds to the daily total.

The World Health Organization guidelines for physical activity[4] recommend a minimum of 150 minutes per week of moderate-intensity activity like brisk walking, biking or dancing... or 75 minutes a week of vigorous activity like jogging or playing an active sport. If you have a chronic disease, check with your doctor first, start slowly and increase activity gradually. You can expect a few sore muscles as you begin, but stop exercising and contact your doctor right away if you experience any chest pain or other alarming symptoms. Any exercise that makes it difficult to speak is likely too intense and could be a risk to your immediate health. Specialized exercise programs are available in some areas to help those with chronic diseases, such as heart disease or back problems, to get started safely.

The cardiac rehab program my husband took after his heart attack in 2004 was a game-changer, and we've worked to keep up our activity level since then. In fact, in 2019 he enrolled in a refresher of this program to bolster his motivation and learn about new recommendations!

Besides the Moving Medicine program in the UK mentioned earlier, Canadian medical schools are also revising their curricula to teach future doctors about the benefits of exercise to prevent and treat chronic diseases. It's better and less costly to prevent diseases than to treat them!

*References:*

Exercise is Medicine, and Doctors are Starting to Prescribe It, The Conversation https://theconversation.com/exercise-is-medicine-and-doctors-are-starting-to-prescribe-it-104390

Prescribing Movement (UK website to encourage doctors to prescribe exercise) https://movingmedicine.ac.uk/

Girls and Women Need More Time in Nature to be Healthy https://theconversation.com/girls-and-women-need-more-time-in-nature-to-be-healthy-104464

Worldwide Trends in Physical Inactivity 2001-2016 https://www.thelancet.com/journals/langlo/article/PIIS2214-109X(18)30357-7/fulltexttbl2

# What can we learn from other cultures?

Now that we're retired, my husband and I like to spend a few months in Spain in the winter (barring any pandemics, of course!). I'm quite fascinated by several distinct differences in culture and lifestyle between Spain and North America—differences that could affect health—some positive and some not-so-positive!

First, I've noticed that people use public transit much more than we do in most areas of Canada and the US. Streets in old European cities are extremely narrow (many cars have dents!), and parking is hard to find and often expensive. We've seen cars parked in the strangest places...

Many city apartments simply don't have parking, leaving tenants with cars to park on the street, wherever they can find a place. The old section of Marbella, where we have stayed in the past, actually allows only delivery vehicles in the narrow streets. We had to pull our suitcases along cobbled walkways to get to our apartment as our taxi had to drop us off outside the Casco Antigua de Marbella (the Old City of Marbella)!

Besides the obvious decrease in pollution from car exhaust, though, using public transit means you are walking a lot more—even if it's just to the bus stop, and then from the stop to your destination. This can build a significant amount of exercise into your day, without needing to think about it.

Cities in Europe are often more densely populated, and every neighbourhood has its grocery store, bakery, fish shop etc. so you can easily walk to do your errands. Many people, especially the elderly, have shopping bags on wheels to take their purchases home easily, pulling them behind as they walk. Neighbourhood stores are busy because many people live nearby and support the convenient local shops. It seems like cities are organized to make cars unnecessary and unwanted!

This contrasts with home and with North American vacations we've taken, where it's too far to walk to any type of shopping. While our winter weather in Canada and the northern US encourages us to use cars more, we often have only a few large grocery stores that serve an entire city rather than many smaller local neighbourhood shops within walking distance. The result is, we drive everywhere rather than fitting our exercise into our daily routine, then we need to add in exercise time. Sometimes we even pay to get some exercise!

Of course, the stretch of land on the southern coast of Spain, the Costa del Sol, is so beautiful with the Mediterranean on one side and the mountains that block the cold northern winds, creating a warmer climate, on the other. We enjoy simply wandering around, soaking up the beauty of the area, people watching and sight seeing—sometimes we don't realize how much walking we're doing. We've visited several neighbouring cities, travelling there by bus, and spent the entire day walking... often up hills and small mountains, then back down again, of course!

The tourism offices have been very helpful in sorting out bus schedules and stops, and we have had no problems getting where we want to go. Choosing a vacation in a place like Spain, with comfortable temperatures that encourage you to be outside walking all day, may mean you will go home in better physical shape than you were when you arrived. I know we have!

Another interesting tradition in Spain is the siesta—many stores close in the afternoon for several hours. I still haven't figured out whether the siesta time is the same for all businesses, but have caught myself walking to a store to make a purchase, only to find them closed. But the siesta gives them time to relax, spend time with family, and eat a healthy mid-day meal while still being open for the busiest parts of the workday. Mid-afternoon is also the hottest time of day and probably the quietest for business.

However, if you really need an item, it's best to head out shopping early in the morning. Better signs with hours of operation would certainly help visitors to accommodate, but regular customers seem to have adjusted to the system with no problems. The siesta is such a long-standing tradition that many stores don't post the hours they open and close in the afternoon—only posting the morning opening and the evening closing times–while other stores catering to tourists no longer take part in the traditional siesta at all, and just stay open. But this tradition is all about lifestyle and is good for workers, especially those who are running a small business themselves and trying to offer service to morning shoppers as well as the evening crowd.

On the "downside", I am amazed at how many Europeans, especially young people, still smoke. It's made me realize policies that ban smoking in restaurants, vehicles and in public places make a difference in how acceptable it is to smoke, effectively "de-normalizing" it in North America. In areas of Europe we've visited, it's normal to see people smoking everywhere. It seems strange compared to Canada, where the activity is banned in so many public places. It is easy to see that passing these types of laws, making smoking much less acceptable, results in fewer smokers overall and certainly decreases exposure to second-hand smoke that has been shown to affect the health of non-smokers. While actual smoking rates are lower in the US and Canada (approximately 16-17%) compared to Spain and France (at 24%) and even higher in northern Europe, the additional difference of being allowed to smoke in public places makes smoking appear even more prevalent.[5]

So, this is what I've learned from my experiences vacationing in Europe (besides some Spanish and French): building activity into every day, rather than thinking of activity as a "task" that you need to find time for, may be a better approach to staying fit. The design of cities and neighbourhoods, and the laws we pass (like those for restrictions on smoking) can make a difference in the behaviours and the health of the entire population. Comparing lifestyles in different countries can help us gain new perspectives and ideas to incorporate into our own communities, helping to create a healthier population.

# What does wellness really mean?

The World Health Organization defines wellness as: *"a state of complete physical, mental, and social well-being, and not merely the absence of disease or infirmity."*

However, when I search the internet, I see two types of "wellness" sites:

- Information on wellness (sometimes referred to as lower case "wellness") ... solid advice on ways to promote health and prevent illness, backed by scientific evidence. It includes good nutrition, exercise, sleep, stress reduction and more, and essentially means the opposite of illness.
- Promotional material on Wellness Products (Wellness with a capital "W") ... products often making pseudo-scientific health claims with sketchy proof and often marketed with a high price tag! The Wellness business is a billion-dollar industry...

How can you tell the difference when you're reading a web page? I use two simple ways:

**Who posted the information?**

Is the web page associated with a large health organization, government, or university? The goal of these organizations is often to share information and promote public health. They have no financial incentive to hide negative information or exaggerate the positive effects of a wellness strategy.

Does the author have any credentials or experience as a health professional? While credentials are not entirely necessary (a talented reporter will get all the facts and present them unbiasedly), it means they will probably have better background knowledge.

Look for references. Where did the information originate? Is it backed by scientific studies? A well referenced web page will have links to background studies that support what they are saying so you can easily find and read the source of the information yourself. Studies usually have a summary at the beginning, called an "abstract" that is a brief description of the study. I also look at where the information was published—many large medical organizations publish journals with information for their members that is usually well researched.

With that in mind, although some knowledge in this book comes from my personal and professional experience as a pharmacist of 40 years, I have shared reputable sources to confirm the information I include here.

**Who paid for it?**

The second thing I look for on a web page is who paid to publicize the information, and whose advertising is displayed with the article. I learned an excellent lesson over 25 years ago when the internet was just starting. The doctors next door asked if I could supply them with information about the herbal medicine, St. John's Wort. I quickly found an article that looked perfect on the internet. My pharmacy student, who was more tech-savvy than me, didn't say a word. She just scrolled down and pointed to the advertisement for St. John's Wort. It was a page designed to sell a product... An "aha" moment for me!

With a more critical look, I noticed the site described the herb as "safer than aspirin". While many would interpret this as saying it is very safe, as a pharmacist, I know that aspirin can cause internal bleeding in some people. The site wasn't being open and honest in an attempt to increase sales. Chances were good they were hiding other important, but negative, information. I subscribed to an independent herbal website after that so I could easily access unbiased information about natural medicines.

So, whether your reason for looking for wellness information or alternative medicines is wanting to stay healthy as you age, or to address a need that is unmet by the medical system, don't be taken in by marketing strategies for Wellness products. Know that a vitamin is a vitamin—they are all the same chemical structure—so there is no reason to pay $90 for a month's supply when you can always buy good quality vitamins from a reputable manufacturer at your local pharmacy for much less. When looking for health information on the internet, choose an academic or health-center site rather than one sponsored by a product manufacturer. Know when you're being marketed to and be a savvy shopper.

But also make sure any alternative treatment is an addition to good medical care and not a replacement for it. Consider natural treatments as complementary to your medical treatment rather than a true "alternative". Nothing can replace good medical care.

So, talk to your doctor or pharmacist about any non-prescription medications you are taking, even if they are being recommended by another health professional. Your family doctor can be an "overseer" of your health, ensuring that all medications you take and health strategies you are using are working together to keep you healthy. While they may not have learned about natural medicines in medical school, they can help you evaluate the information you are reading and ensure there is no interference with any health condition you may have. Your pharmacist may be your most accessible health professional, and they can help ensure you avoid conflicts with medications you are already taking. They also have access to scientific references on alternative and complementary products. Ask if they can find some solid information to share with you and, if necessary, with your doctor.

Talking with your doctor and pharmacist about non-prescription choices is also a great way to start a conversation around your health goals and how best to achieve them. The internet can be a wonderful source of information, but it's best when used in consultation with your doctors, pharmacists, and other health professionals.

*References:*

The Self-Care Paradox https://elemental.medium.com/the-self-care-paradox-1480eaf72977

# Does a better attitude help?

**Ever heard the saying: Life is short, eat dessert first?**

Does life seem too short? When you look back, will you be happy with what you've accomplished? Are there things you've always wanted to do but just can't find the time to get started? Do you sometimes feel like you should eat dessert first in case your mealtime is cut short?

**Where does the time go?**

Despite our current hurried lifestyles with their many distractions and demands on our time, this isn't a recent problem. I stumbled across an essay entitled "On the Shortness of Life" by Roman philosopher, Lucius Annaeus Seneca, written almost 2000 years ago. Even back then, people complained that life was too short. Though the average lifespan is years longer now, most of us still feel the same.

In his essay, Seneca wrote, "our lifetime offers ample scope to the person who maps it out well... It's not that we have a short time to live, but that we waste much of it. Men are thrifty in guarding their private property, but as soon as it comes to wasting time, they are most extravagant with the one commodity for which it's respectable to be greedy. No one values time: all use it more than lavishly, as if it cost nothing." With time, once it's gone you can't get it back...

**So, how do you "map it out well" as Seneca suggests?**

You may have heard of the 80/20 rule: 80% of benefit often comes from 20% of your effort. Keeping this in mind, if we became purposeful and productive with just 20% of our time, we might still reap 80% of the benefit we achieve in a normal unstructured day. It's difficult to change your entire life, but what about just 20% of it? Or even 10%?

**Here's one way to do it...**

<u>First:</u> Take some time to decide what you really want from life. What are your most important goals that you've not yet achieved? What have you always wanted to do that you haven't yet tried? Have you developed relationships you value? Interviews with dying patients suggest regrets are often focused on things they haven't made time to do, or relationships they neglected to develop with important people in their lives. These are areas where you want to focus; these are things you want create time to do now. But keep in mind that your goals will probably change over time, and you will want to reassess and refocus some time down the road...

<u>Second:</u> Ask yourself: Are you working on these goals that are important to you or just keeping "busy" with life? Remember the 80/20 rule and carve some time away for yourself from activities that really don't matter in the overall picture. Use this time to focus on what is really important to you.

<u>Third:</u> Don't multitask. Turn off distractions so you can increase your efficiency to accomplish more in this limited amount of special time you've created for yourself. Multitasking lowers the quality of your attention, makes you tire faster, increases your stress and unhappiness, and lessens the effectiveness of your activity or learning.

**Start now...**

I've always been a procrastinator... in fact, my parents once gave me a little round medallion with the letters "TUIT" engraved on it—"I'll do it when I get around to it" (a round TUIT)... a little family joke. My dad also used to call me "the late Jeannie Collins" because I was late so often, having been oblivious to time and put off preparing to go somewhere! So, learn from my lazy choices...

When we first spent an entire winter in Florida, I had several retirement activities that I wanted to do... things I'd been wanting to try, like improving my drawing, trying some painting and learning a new language. As the winter passed and March rolled around, I realized that I'd put off starting these activities, day after day, thinking that I had lots of time to get around to it. I'd "wasted" 4 months of what I thought would be a long "empty" winter! It was so easy to just fill in the time with other interesting activities.

Knowing I only had 2 more months left there, helped me to focus on what was important to me at the time—the things I really wanted to do—and I was able to accomplish a lot. The ancient Roman, Seneca, also said, "The greatest waste of life lies in postponement: it robs us of each day in turn and snatches away the present by promising the future." At some point, like me, you need to decide to get started and do the things you really want to do. The alternative, truly, is just giving up on your dreams.

I started setting some time aside every day for what was important to me. At least I made good use of the last 2 months I was there to achieve a few things I'd always wanted to do. I really enjoyed learning how to draw portraits and became quite good at it with the time I spent practicing.

So, remember that the most common regrets expressed at the end of life are not about what the person did, but about what they wanted to do but never found (or made) the time for. So, what can you do to make sure this isn't one of your regrets? Just as you can choose to be happy, decide now to accomplish (or at least work on) your life's greatest desires. Consciously making choices now can help you experience satisfaction and happiness as you go through life and when you look back on your past.

"Eating dessert first", of course, isn't really talking about food... Many of us think of dessert as the tastiest, most desirable part of a meal. The "life" version of dessert refers to the best, most fun, and most rewarding parts of life. The expression is encouraging us to save time for what could be the best parts of our lives. The decisions you make about what you'll do today can change your future.


*References:*

Why you don't need to read those productivity guides https://medium.com/the-polymath-project/why-you-dont-need-to-read-those-productivity-guides-347fe02cc196

Seneca, on the greatest obstacle to living a more fulfilling life https://medium.com/personal-growth/ seneca-on-the-greatest-obstacle-to-living-a-more-fulfilling-life-ce0a6521494d

On the Shortness of Life, Seneca. Full text (translated) https://archive.org/ stream/SenecaOnTheShortnessOfLife/ Seneca+on+the+Shortness+of+Life_djvu.txt

# Chapter 2: What if I Have Stomach Problems?

## Do you take daily stomach medicine?

If you have been taking potent acid-suppressing drugs [Losec (Prilosec in the USA), Nexxium, Prevacid, Tecta, Dexilant or others] regularly for over 8 weeks, talk to your doctor about whether you should continue taking them. Although recommended long-term for some conditions, recent studies have found that 40 to 55% of people are taking them for no diagnosed reason.

One factor that keeps people on these drugs, known as PPI's (Proton Pump Inhibitors), is that many people experience "rebound hyperacidity", or increased production of stomach acid, when they stop the medication. So, when you stop these drugs after prolonged treatment, you can expect a worsening of your symptoms simply because you stopped the medication. New guidelines are available to help your doctor advise you how to quit these medications if they are no longer needed.

Although this class of acid-reducing drugs has been available for over 25 years and is generally regarded as safe, with some being sold now without prescription, some problems have been associated with long-term daily use. Here are some examples:

- Decreased absorption of some vitamins and minerals that need stomach acid for absorption (calcium, magnesium, vitamin B12 and possibly iron, and vitamin C).

- Decreased bone density (due to decreased absorption of calcium) with associated increase in fractures of the wrist, hip and spine.

- Increased muscle spasms (due to decreased magnesium)

- Interactions with some drugs (clopidogrel [Plavix, taken to prevent blood clots], high-dose methotrexate [used to treat cancer]).

• Increased growth of certain unfavourable bacteria in the digestive system (C. difficile, Traveller's Diarrhea, Small Intestine Bacterial Overgrowth).

• Increase risk of developing pneumonia (likely associated with increased bacteria in the digestive system).

"Observational" studies suggest an association of use of PPI drugs with increased cancers of the esophagus and stomach, dementia, chronic kidney disease and heart attacks. Although observational studies do not prove the drugs cause these conditions, they establish an association, and this has created some concerns. The drugs ,are recommended for preventing acid reflux in patients with Barrett's Esophagus (scar tissue in the esophagus caused by long-term acid reflux, believed to be a precursor for cancer of the esophagus); however, one study observed increased rates of cancer in patients who took PPI's daily. Hopefully, future studies will be done to determine whether these drugs are truly a cause of the observed increased risk. Meanwhile, they should be taken only when clearly needed.

Changing the acidity of the stomach long-term also affects what types of bacteria flourish there, both harmful and non-harmful. And we know stomach acid is a protective agent in preventing harmful organisms entering our bodies.

A newly reported study done at the University of Southern California has suggested a mechanism for multiple organ damage from acid suppressing drugs. PPI drugs block the pumping mechanism that pumps acids into the stomach, but they found these drugs also block similar acid pumps in the tiny enzymatic "garbage disposal" lysosome sacks within other cells in the body, reducing the acid they need to function. This, they propose, allows waste to build up inside cells in the kidney, brain and lining of blood vessels, causing cells to age more quickly and dysfunction. This could explain how drugs designed to dramatically reduce acid in the stomach could affect other organs. However, more research is needed—so far, this is just a theory, although an interesting one.

Meanwhile, many people are taking these drugs for no documented reason and others may do just as well on a lower level acid suppressing drug such as a Histamine-2 Receptor Antagonist (H2RA) [for example, ranitidine (Zantac) and famotidine (Pepcid)] that don't have these side effects.

The guidelines recommend lowering the daily dose, stopping, switching to "as needed" use, or changing to an H2RA to reduce acid, once a person has completed a course of 4 to 8 weeks to heal an ulcer or esophagus damage from heartburn. Note that "rebound hypersecretion" of acid can occur for up to 2 weeks when long-term PPI drugs are discontinued, and this is difficult to distinguish from the original problem. Reducing the dose gradually and introducing non-drug strategies (diet/lifestyle changes) may help reduce symptoms on discontinuation of PPI's.

The detailed deprescribing guideline recommendations are available in the footnote below[6].

# Stomach meds and Lupus...

A new report in our Canadian pharmacy journal, Pharmacy Practice Plus, described a Health Canada review of the association between stomach medications known as Proton Pump Inhibitors (or PPIs) and a type of autoimmune disease, SCLE (Subacute Cutaneous Lupus Erythematosis). They determined that there was enough evidence of an association between the drugs and this disease that manufacturers needed to update product safety information to include this discovery.

SCLE is a rare disease, but since PPI drugs are available without prescription and so many people take them regularly, Health Canada wants to raise awareness of this potential safety issue. Of 18 international case reports of patients with SCLE taking one of several PPI medications, 16 recovered when they stopped the drug, and at least one developed the disease again when they restarted it.

Autoimmune disorders have increased worldwide in Westernized societies over the past 30 years. Currently it is estimated that approximately 2 million Canadians and up to 23.5 million Americans suffer from autoimmune diseases, such as Lupus, Type 1 diabetes, inflammatory bowel diseases, MS, Rheumatoid Arthritis, and Hashimoto's Thyroiditis (the main cause of low thyroid)... all are caused by an immune system not working properly. Although studies are scarce, in the US immune disorders were documented to have risen from 3% of the population in the 1960s to 9% in 2009.

Given that bacteria in the gut are now known to influence the immune system, and that PPIs can cause a change in gut bacteria, it should not be a surprise that there is an association between their use and an autoimmune disease. Perhaps researchers should look at whether there might be an association between PPIs and other diseases caused by immune system dysfunction.

If you have an autoimmune disease and are taking regular stomach medications, talk to your doctor about this association and whether you should stop your stomach medication.

# Chapter 3: Are Herbal (Natural) Medications Safe to Take?

## Natural Medications

Many people think that herbal medications, being natural, are completely safe to take. But this isn't always true. Herbal medications are really medicines, but just still in their natural plant form. Some are safer than others.

A new study, published in January 2018 in the British Journal of Clinical Pharmacology, analyzed severe reactions between herbs and drugs that were reported in journals as clinical studies or case reports. They looked at which drugs and diseases were most commonly involved, and how severe the reactions were.

They found interactions of varying types. Herbs could either increase the rate at which regular medications were removed from the body resulting in too little medication, or they could slow down the clearance, leaving too much of the medication left in the person's system. This could cause patients to respond poorly to their prescription medication or to develop toxic reactions to their regular treatments. Either scenario could result in hospitalization for the patient, especially with certain medications.

The most common serious interactions occurred in people who had heart disease, cancer, and kidney transplants. The most common prescription medications affected were the blood thinner warfarin, certain "alkylating" chemotherapy drugs, and the anti-rejection drug, cyclosporin. For each of these drugs, there is a very narrow "treatment window"—getting just a little too much or too little of the drug they need could cause serious problems with their condition.

Many herbal medicines "thin" the blood (i.e. make it less likely for a clot to form) so can add to the effect of warfarin and other anticoagulant or "blood thinner" drugs. Too much thinning of the blood can mean a minor bump to the skin could cause extensive bleeding, seen as bruising. Worse, the bleeding can sometimes happen inside the body, usually in the digestive system, where it can't easily be seen, leading to significant blood loss. One sign that shows a person is losing blood in the digestive system is a black, "tarry" stool - by the time blood reaches the end of the digestive system, it has turned from red to a sticky black, and looks much like tar.

Warfarin works by blocking the production of substances made from vitamin K that the body uses to make a blood clot. Many plants contain vitamin K, including herbal medicines. Increasing the amount of vitamin K in the diet, whether as a green leafy food or a herbal medicine, can help the body make more vitamin K clotting agents—more for the warfarin to block—requiring a higher dose of warfarin to prevent clots. In other words, more vitamin K can suddenly mean the blood will clot more easily, increasing the risk of a blood clot, the underlying cause of heart attacks and most strokes.

Both chemotherapy drugs and cyclosporin, the anti-rejections drug, need to be given in exact amounts to work properly. Too little and they don't work as well... too much and they become toxic. So even a slight change in how quickly they are cleared from the body can result in too much or too little in the system. Any person taking these medications should check a reputable source of information before taking a herbal medicine—ideally their doctor or pharmacist.

Pharmacists receive education in both herbal and standard medications as part of their training. They have access to information on diseases, drugs, herbals, and interactions between these. If you take any prescription medications and are considering starting a herbal medicine, check with your pharmacist first. However, realize that a thorough information search requires time. If possible, leave the question with your pharmacist and drop back later to allow time for a proper search.

As well, herbals can interact with a medical condition you have. For example, blood sugar levels can be affected by some herbal medicines and this can be significant if you have diabetes. So, be sure to ask about interactions with both medications you take and any medical conditions you have.

Doctors and pharmacists recommend keeping a list of all your medications for emergency use. But, as you can see, it is equally important to include all supplements you take on your list. Many pharmacies now provide a printed list that is automatically updated each time you fill a prescription. If you take any herbal medicine or nutritional supplement regularly, ask your pharmacist to add these to your profile so their information—and your list—will be complete. And, having complete information in their computer system, means the computer will bring possible interactions to the pharmacist's attention every time they fill a prescription. Lastly, share your list with all health professionals who give you treatment... it just might prevent an avoidable interaction!

## Everything In Moderation...

Medications, prescription and natural ones, can relief discomfort, treat diseases and even save lives. But they can also have side effects and interact with each other or with health conditions you have. With medications, "less is more". You always want to be taking the lowest dose of the fewest medications that will achieve your health goals.

# Chapter 4: How Can I Prevent Heart Disease and Stroke?

## How Important is Blood Cholesterol?

Did you know there is a controversy over whether low-density cholesterol (LDL-cholesterol, also referred to as "bad cholesterol") actually causes heart disease or is simply a secondary effect of the true cause? I didn't until I stumbled across an article by researchers at several Japanese universities...

This research article, written by independent university researchers in Japan, examined cholesterol levels and longevity, and reported that increased blood cholesterol was correlated to a longer life span in the elderly—the opposite to what we would expect if high cholesterol is bad for our health and causes cardiovascular disease (including heart attacks and strokes). This study, entitled "Towards a Paradigm Shift in Cholesterol Treatment", is available at the link in the footnote below[7], if you are interested in reading it yourself.

Having studied hormones for many years, I know our bodies make hormones from cholesterol. Cholesterol is also used to make vitamin D and bile (a fluid produced by the liver and used to digest and absorb fat), and it is a component of the walls of our cells.

We get cholesterol from our food, and our liver also produces it. When we eat more cholesterol, our liver produces less, and when we eat less, the liver makes more, attempting to keep the blood level constant. Our bodies do this with many essential nutrients, like calcium, magnesium, iron, sugar, etc. storing away, pulling from storage sites or producing as necessary to maintain the blood levels our bodies need to function. This is known as "homeostasis". Cholesterol is one of these essential molecules that our bodies try to keep at a constant level. The only way to lower cholesterol significantly is to take medication.

As a pharmacist, I have seen many reports of studies over the years that, I believed, proved the cholesterol/heart disease theory without question. Through my professional education, I learned that high cholesterol, especially LDL-cholesterol, in the blood was a major cause of plaques that block arteries carrying essential blood to the heart muscle, and that lowering cholesterol would reduce the risk of a heart attack and result in a longer lifespan. I counselled patients to reduce their intake of animal fat and increase their consumption of "good" polyunsaturated fats, such as the omega-3 oils, as I had been taught.

Now that I'm retired and have more time to read, and with my interest piqued by the article I stumbled across, I started looking more closely at the research... I was shocked at what I found!

I found articles from researchers in several areas of the world that questioned cholesterol as a cause of heart disease. A text by Uffe Ravnskov, entitled "The Cholesterol Myths", seemed to cover the controversy well, describing flaws in several studies that were interpreted to support the diet/cholesterol/heart disease theory. Dr. Ravnskov is a family physician, now retired, who noted that this new idea didn't seem to agree with information he had previously learned when training as a physician. He examined the original full version of studies used to support this idea and found what he believed were flaws. He continued reading related research and found several other studies that appeared to conflict with the idea that dietary fat and cholesterol cause heart disease. He began writing articles and eventually wrote a book on his findings.

The original 1998 version of the book is available free online[8] and you can ask for the updated version at your favourite bookstore. It certainly is an interesting read.

Ravnskov begins with discussing the original study by Dr. Ancel Keyes in 1953 that started us into the world of low-fat diets and cholesterol medications. This study used data from six countries that clearly showed higher fat in the diet resulted in higher rates of heart disease. But data were available from 22 countries at the time, and when all countries were included, the association was not clear at all. Some countries with similar dietary fat to that in the US actually had only 1/3 to 1/4 the rate of heart related deaths but he did not include these in his assessment. He cherry-picked his countries to make a graph that best supported his idea. A scientific publication should never do this.

Ravnskov also describes several studies of populations with high cholesterol and high-fat diets that have very low heart disease rates, and populations within the same country, where the affluent have much higher rates of heart disease than the poor, but where blood cholesterol and genetics would be similar on average.

According to the "Scientific Method", the basis of all scientific study, the original hypothesis or theory must be re-evaluated whenever any consistent conflicting study results are found. While the "statin" cholesterol medications (the type most commonly used currently) have been shown to reduce heart disease deaths, they have many actions in the body other than simply lowering LDL cholesterol that could benefit those at risk of heart disease. There is enough conflicting evidence that the benefit versus risk of these drugs should be reassessed objectively.

Lack of physical activity, mental stress, smoking and obesity are all considered risk factors for heart disease and stroke. These factors also increase the level of cholesterol in the blood. If the blood cholesterol level is merely secondary to the actual causes of heart disease, then artificially lowering it without changing the underlying sedentary lifestyle, stress, smoking and overweight would have little effect on reducing heart disease risk. If this is the case, we need to re-evaluate our focus on LDL-cholesterol and place more importance on changing lifestyle factors that are associated with increased risk.

However, cholesterol medications known as "statins" (their names end with -statin) do more than just lower cholesterol. They also reduce inflammation, act as an antioxidant, and "thin" the blood ("anti-coagulant" action)–actions that help reduce the risk of heart disease. Is it possible that these are the actions that give protection from heart disease, rather than the cholesterol-lowering effect? Given that earlier cholesterol drugs had little effect on actual rates of cardiovascular deathsth, this is possible. But, to my knowledge, this has not been investigated. One reference suggests: "It may be wiser to search for the lowest effective dose instead of the dose with maximal effect on LDL-cholesterol."

I am certainly not advising anyone to stop taking their medication, and lowering cholesterol in those under age 47 who have inherited high cholesterol (called *familial hypercholesterolemia)* has well proven benefit, but my question is: Should we be focusing more on the factors that raise cholesterol and less on trying to lower our cholesterol numbers artificially? A new study (PURE—Prospective Urban Rural Epidemiology study) and newer cardiovascular guidelines put less emphasis on cholesterol and more on blood pressure, diabetes and other risk factors for heart disease. Study authors concluded: "Focusing on a single lipid marker such as LDL cholesterol alone does not capture the net clinical effects of nutrients on cardiovascular risk."

In an interview, one study author also said, "My advice to the general population is to lead a healthy lifestyle. Don't smoke and take exercise — those two things are clearly beneficial. And then I would say maintain a reasonable weight. You don't want to be too overweight, but you also don't want to be too skinny. Eat a balanced diet — a bit of meat, fish, several portions of fruit and vegetables, but you don't have to be vegan or eat an excessive amount of plants to be healthy."

Senior author of the PURE study, Dr Salim Yusuf (McMaster University, Hamilton, ON) commented: "This is good old-fashioned advice. When I showed these results to my mother, she said, 'Why did you bother doing this study? This is what our grandmothers and their grandmothers have been advocating for centuries.' And actually she is right." Interesting quote!

If you are taking medications for cholesterol, discuss this information with your doctor, encourage him or her to examine the evidence and discuss it with local specialists, and thoroughly review possible adverse effects of your medication to ensure you receive more benefit than risk from what you are taking. While newer guidelines for preventing cardiovascular disease still recommend lowering cholesterol, it is being given less importance and more emphasis is put on other strategies such as increasing activity, reducing stress and quitting smoking to reduce cardiovascular risk. Keep a focus on continuing to improve your lifestyle in these areas, whether or not you take medication.

Following the scientific method of study, the basis of current research, we constantly need to question the status quo when additional evidence comes to light. This is how we continually improve the quality of our healthcare and our health.

*References:*

<u>PURE Shakes Up Nutritional Field: Finds High Fat Intake [1]Beneficial (medscape.com)[2]</u>

---

1. https://www.medscape.com/viewarticle/884937

2. https://www.medscape.com/viewarticle/884937

# Is Controlling Blood Pressure Important?

There's almost always a discussion about your blood pressure when you visit your doctor, but how much do you really know about it? Here are a few facts to help you understand why it's important, how to monitor your pressure and some things you can do to keep it healthy...

**What is blood pressure?**

Blood pressure is a measure of the pressure inside your arteries. This pressure increases and decreases with each heartbeat. Your heart pumps out blood with each beat, with enough pressure to send it through the arteries to all parts of the body. This pressure drops between each heartbeat, while the heart relaxes and refills with blood. Your doctor or nurse measures the highest and lowest pressure for each beat, called the "systolic" and "diastolic" measurements.

Blood pressure changes constantly. Exercise, caffeine, smoking, anxiety, stress, and even a full bladder can raise your blood pressure. Relaxing can lower it.

# What can high blood pressure do?

Uncontrolled high blood pressure is the number one risk factor for stroke and an important risk factor for heart disease. It can also cause damage to various organs.

<u>Damage to arteries</u>

Under constant high pressure, the inner lining of blood vessels can become damaged and inflamed, allowing fats in the bloodstream to collect in the lining. These fatty areas also collect deposits of calcium and are called "plaque". They can stiffen and eventually block an artery, or they can burst open and cause a blood clot to form, instantly blocking the artery. Some researchers have suggested plaque formation may be the body's way of protecting and healing damaged areas, somewhat like a scab does on the outside of the body, but this is yet to be proven.

Over time, with constant pressure, a section of artery wall can also become weakened and bulge outward. This is called an aneurysm and, if it bursts, it can cause life-threatening bleeding inside the body. Aneurysms can form in any artery, but they're most dangerous when they develop in the brain or on the aorta, the body's largest artery that runs from the left side of the heart down into the abdomen.

<u>Damage to the heart</u>

When blood pressure is high, your heart must work harder to pump blood against this increased pressure. Over time, the left side of the heart that pumps blood through the body can become larger and stiffen because of the extra work it needs to do. This limits the heart's ability to supply the body with enough blood and to keep up with the blood returning to the heart from the lungs. We call this heart failure (also known as cardiac insufficiency) and it also increases your risk of a heart attack.

<u>Damage to the brain</u>

A stroke occurs when part of the brain is deprived of blood, causing brain cells to die. Uncontrolled high blood pressure can damage blood vessels in the brain, causing them to narrow, burst or leak. It can also cause blood clots to form in the arteries leading to the brain, blocking blood flow and potentially causing a stroke.

Reduced blood flow to the brain can also cause dementia, a result of gradual damage to areas of the brain that control thinking, speaking, decision-making, memory, vision and movement.

<u>Damage to eyes and kidneys</u>

Both the eyes and kidneys contain tiny blood vessels that can become damaged, leading to vision problems and kidney failure.

**What is a good blood pressure?**

- Ideal—120/80

- Normal—less than 140/90

- Exceptions:

- Diabetes—best if less than 130/80

- Over 80 years—less than 150 Diastolic (higher number)

Low blood pressure (less than 120/80) is fine unless it is low enough to make you dizzy or lightheaded. A doctor once told me having naturally low blood pressure was "like having extra insurance".

# What can you do to control blood pressure?

We can't control some risk factors, such as age, ethnicity, and gender. After age 65, women are more likely than men to develop high blood pressure. Pregnancy, birth control, and menopause can also increase the chance of developing high blood pressure.

But there is plenty you can do:

- Eat a healthy diet. Learn about the DASH diet (Dietary Approaches to Stop Hypertension) at the link below[9], an eating plan designed to help lower high blood pressure. This diet includes healthy foods and limits salt intake.

- Be active for at least 150 minutes per week, at least 10 minutes at a time.

- Maintain a healthy body weight. If overweight, losing even 5% to 10% of your weight can help lower blood pressure and reduce risk of heart attack or stroke.

- Don't smoke!

- Limit alcohol to 2 drinks a day/10 per week for women, and 3 per day/15 per week for men.

- Find healthy ways to manage your stress.

**How to measure blood pressure at home**

1. Read and follow the specific instructions for your monitor, then follow these general instructions:
2. Relax in a quiet area for 5 to 10 minutes.
3. Slide the cuff on your arm with lower edge about 1 inch above elbow fold. Fasten snugly but not too tight (you should be able to slide 2 fingers underneath).

4. Sit up straight, back against the chair, legs uncrossed, arm resting on the table, palm up. Relax and don't talk during the measurement.
5. If using an automatic monitor, press the button now. If not, continue with steps below:
6. Inflate the cuff about 30 points higher than the expected measurement, or until the machine says to stop. (some monitors do the rest automatically).
7. Loosen the airflow valve so that the pressure falls by 2 to 3 points with each heartbeat.
8. With a manual (stethoscope) monitor, listen for the first pulse (heartbeat) sound.
    a. Note the reading on the gauge/screen
    b. This is the upper (systolic) reading
9. Continue to deflate the cuff slowly
    a. Listen until the heartbeat sound disappears
    b. This is the lower (diastolic) reading
10. Let the cuff completely deflate. Remove the cuff.
11. Repeat this twice, resting for several minutes between readings. Use the lowest reading.
12. Record the date, time, and lowest measurement. Bring the records to your doctor's visits. Once a year, bring your machine to check its accuracy by comparing with your doctor's reading. Your doctor, nurse or pharmacist can also check your technique.

So, yes, high blood pressure is important to control. Uncontrolled, it can quietly damage your body over a period of years—they call it the "Silent killer". So, have your doctor check your blood pressure regularly, or check it yourself. Take action if your pressure is consistently increased to prevent blood pressure complications.

**References:**

High Blood Pressure (Heart and Stroke Association) https://www.heartandstroke.ca/heart/risk-and-prevention/condition-risk-factors/high-blood-pressure

Checking Your Blood Pressure at Home (WebMD) https://www.webmd.com/hypertension-high-blood-pressure/guide/hypertension-home-monitoring1-4

High blood pressure dangers (Mayo Clinic) https://www.mayoclinic.org/diseases-conditions/high-blood-pressure/in-depth/high-blood-pressure/art-20045868

# Chapter 5: Are Microbes in Our Gut Important?

## Gut Microbes

We humans, each of us, have trillions of microbes that live inside and on the surface of our bodies—most experts say about 3 to 4 pounds' worth. These include over 10,000 different types of microbes (including bacteria, viruses, and fungi), collectively known as our "microbiome". And having a larger variety of microbes in our system may protect us against future illness—new research suggests they give us resilience against disease.

For many years we only heard about bad bacteria, viruses and fungi that cause disease. But most organisms are beneficial, and, in fact, we can't live without them. We need to think of these good microscopic inhabitants of our bodies as a part of us we need to keep healthy. We have a "symbiotic" relationship: we evolved together and rely on each other for survival.

The pharmacy school at the University of Toronto hosted an online Town Hall Medicine summit on the microbiome where 21 researchers spoke about results of research they have been conducting in this area. I listened to most of the lectures and want to share some of what I learned with you. The series is still available (for a fee) if you are interested in learning more. It's available at the link below.[10]

**What do microbes do for us?**

These microorganisms perform many bodily functions for us: from helping to digest our food and absorb nutrients, to protecting us from disease, to controlling how our immune system functions, and more. Although they've been researching our microbiome for over 10 years, scientists are still learning how they interact with our human cells with significant increases in understanding in the last 5 years. They now believe the make-up and health of the microbiome can affect obesity, autism, allergies, intestinal health, responses to drugs, rheumatoid arthritis, Type 1 diabetes and many other conditions.

Inflammatory diseases, like Multiple Sclerosis (MS), asthma and Crohn's disease, have been on the rise over the past 50 years. Researchers have proposed the "hygiene theory" which suggests that decreased exposure to microbes, through overuse of antibacterial agents and just being too clean, has led to decreased diversity of our bodies' beneficial microbes. Some evidence suggests that exposure to good bacteria in the early years of life is crucial to avoid inflammatory diseases, such as asthma and inflammatory bowel disease, later in life. Think of it as giving your immune system "exercise" to help it strengthen and learn to function properly.

# The gut and the brain "talk" to each other...

Recently they have even identified communication between gut bacteria and the brain, through hormones, nerves, and chemicals known as neurotransmitters. They believe that this communication affects our mental health. What we eat influences the composition and activity of the microbiome, and this has led to research on how our diet could influence mental health. For example, newer studies suggest eating a western diet of highly processed food may increase risk of depression and anxiety. But choosing a Mediterranean diet, with higher amounts of vegetables and good fats like olive oil, may reduce risk of these mood disorders. This field of study is called nutritional psychiatry.

We also have a major nerve, called the vagus, that directly connects the brain and the gut. Years ago, surgeons would sometimes cut this nerve in patients who had ulcers caused by stress. The ulcers healed, but many patients developed psychiatric problems afterward. It turns out that this nerve is a two-way street, carrying messages from the gut to the brain as well as in the other direction, and it's another important way our gut and our brain communicate.

I've read about an abdominal breathing technique that is suggested help with relaxation: the belly is pushed out during inhalation and pulled in while exhaling. I'd always thought this was just a distraction technique, a type of meditation to take a person's mind off their troubles. But I've learned that this abdominal movement can stimulate the vagus nerve when done correctly, creating a relaxation response in the brain. Experts stress it requires practice to be able create a full parasympathetic relaxation response that is useful during an episode of stress. However, it seems like a worthwhile skill to develop!

**Exposure early in life is important**

Studies of asthma and allergies are very telling. Children who receive an antibiotic in the first year of life have higher rates of asthma. Studies also suggest growing up on a farm, with a dog, or being born by natural birth versus by sterile caesarean section can create a lower risk for asthma and allergies. These affect the types of bacteria a child is exposed to early in life and therefore will incorporate into their digestive and other systems.

Exposure to organisms in the first 3 years of life—while the immune system is developing—is more important with longer-lasting effects than later in life when our systems are well-established. Trying to repair and maintain a microbiome that is damaged as an adult is more difficult than establishing a healthy one in the first place and requires ongoing effort.

Researchers describe extinction of entire species of microbes in the digestive systems, the "inner world", of some populations. And they can be very difficult to reintroduce permanently, just as it's almost impossible to reintroduce animal species that have become extinct in the outer world. Keep in mind that a typical probiotic capsule contains less than 10 species of organisms, compared to around 10,000 species in a healthy adult. Although probiotics can help, we need to do more.


**How can we help our gut microbes?**

Factors that affect the composition of our microbiome include the food we eat and where we spend our time. With modern urban living, many can spend as much as 90% of their time indoors. Simply spending time in nature can change the organisms we take into our bodies. Bringing fresh fruits, vegetables and plants into the home can help recreate "the farm effect" with benefits to our microbiome.

Eating fermented foods can also help, as the fermentation process creates many beneficial bacteria. One expert recommends five servings per week of at least three different fermented foods. These foods also provide fibre, which feeds good bacteria. Although raw foods contain more live bacteria than those that have been cooked, even organisms killed in the cooking process benefit the immune system.

# Just like a garden...

One expert, Anne Bikle, who is also an avid gardener, describes our large bowel as a "garden" and a "medicine chest", producing substances that protect us from abnormal, potentially cancerous, cells and infections. She tells us that 40% of the compounds in our blood are made by our microbiome, and that we are as much microbial as we are human. She suggests we need to treat our digestive system as we would a garden: feed it plenty of fibre and nutrient rich plants, just as you would add nutrients and compost to soil to have a healthy garden that produces tasty vegetables or beautiful flowers. Her advice in a nutshell? "Mulch your garden soil, inside and out". Keep your inside world <u>and</u> your outside world healthy...

**References:**

Town Hall Medicine, University of Toronto, Leslie Dan Faculty of Pharmacy https://townhallmedicine.com/summit-themes/the-paradigm-shift/ the-beginners-guide-to-the-microbiome/

Are we more microbe than human? https://www.bing.com/ search?q=are+we+more+microbe+than+human&cvid=05b4f6137ab6402f8135af950922bc18&

# Do Gut Microbes Also Affect Arthritis?

Rheumatoid arthritis (RA) is an autoimmune disease where the body's immune system mistakenly attacks itself, causing damage to joints with swelling and pain. It can also cause damage to other parts of the body, including the skin, eyes, heart, lung and blood vessels. To date, no cause or cures have been identified, and treatments focus on relieving pain and swelling, and slowing the progression of the disease.

The Mayo Clinic has reported some interesting research on RA. A study conducted in mice shows a link between the presence of a particular bacterium in the gut, called Collinsella, and increased risk of developing rheumatoid arthritis. This type of bacteria is not usually present in the intestines but was found in significant numbers in people with rheumatoid arthritis, inspiring researchers to run a test in mice.

Researchers infected mice with the Collinsella bacteria, then treated them by introducing a specific good bacterial flora to compete with the unwanted bacteria. This resulted in decreased symptoms and fewer inflammatory indicators associated with rheumatoid arthritis in the treated mice.

Since mice's immune systems and arthritis processes are like those in humans, this suggests that a similar treatment could give people relief from this difficult to treat disease. Further, it suggests that examining intestinal bacteria may provide a way to detect who is at risk of developing arthritis and even the possibility of preventing it from occurring. Researchers expect that, like the mice, humans will be unlikely to experience side effects from this "probiotic" bacteria treatment.

The Mayo Clinic is also researching other autoimmune and infection problems that might be related to improper bacteria in our digestive systems. These include conditions such as

- Gluten sensitivity

- Irritable bowel syndrome

- C. Difficile gut infection

- Colon cancer

- Bacterial vaginosis and

- Other health problems associated with the reproductive system

While it will be interesting to see results of human trials using treatment of RA with good bacteria, there is no reason not to try this therapy on yourself if you are suffering with one of these diseases. Discuss this possibility with your physician!

There are many good quality probiotics available without prescription that might give similar results to the product used in the mice experiment in arthritis. And fermented foods also introduce good bacteria into your digestive system and could be potentially helpful.

This ties in closely with my book review blog post, Bacteria for Breakfast, that discusses how gut bacteria can influence the function of the immune system. Check out my post[11] if you'd like to read more!

Reference: Mayo Clinic Microbiome Program and https://www.ScienceDaily.com/releases/2016/07/160711151315.htm

# Chapter 6: What Does Vitamin K2 Do? Is It Important For Our Health?

## Heart Disease and Osteoporosis are Linked

Who would have thought there could be a connection between heart disease and osteoporosis? I certainly didn't until I read about vitamin K2. The actions of this nutrient, and its unintended reduction in our food supply in North America, may additionally explain why we are seeing too much of these chronic diseases despite all our efforts and complex medications...

The connection is calcium—too little of it leads to thinning of the bones and risk of osteoporosis, and too much can cause calcification (or "hardening") of the arteries. Calcifications, deposits of calcium in the walls of arteries, can cause heart disease when it creates narrowing and blockages in arteries that supply the heart muscle. While this seems to present a paradox... too much calcium in one case and too little in the other... the link is a nutrient that controls where calcium goes in the body.

That nutrient is vitamin K2, a vitamin that was not widely studied until the last 20 years. Its sister vitamin, K1, was researched more thoroughly as it was thought to be the only active form of vitamin K in the body. K1 is needed for blood clotting and is the vitamin whose action is blocked by the blood thinner, warfarin.

Vitamin K2, on the other hand, controls where calcium goes once it's absorbed from the digestive system. It does this by activating two substances: osteocalcin and Matrix GLA Protein (MGP). Once activated by vitamin K2, osteocalcin attracts calcium to bones and teeth, strengthening them. Activated MGP sweeps excess calcium away from soft tissues, including arteries and veins, preventing and removing dangerous plaque from inside arteries. A lack of vitamin K2 means that osteocalcin and MGP cannot be activated and therefore cannot perform these important functions.

Vitamin D is important too. You likely already know that this vitamin is needed to absorb calcium from your digestive system. This makes it an important factor in preventing osteoporosis. You may have taken calcium supplements with vitamin D added right into the tablet and probably have learned that it's called the "sunshine vitamin" because we make it when the sun shines on our skin.

But vitamin D is also needed to make the MGP protein that removes calcium from soft tissues, preventing and reversing hardening of the arteries. So, vitamins D and K2 work together to prevent both osteoporosis and heart disease—vitamin D helps to get calcium into your system, and both vitamins K and D are needed to make sure the calcium goes to the right place.

This information about vitamin K explains several "paradoxes" in our explanation of causes of heart disease: Why do 50% of people who have a heart attack have normal cholesterol? Why do the French, with their rich, fatty diet, have less heart disease than us in North America? (This has been called the "French Paradox"). Why is there so much osteoporosis (a disease of too little calcium) and heart disease (a disease of too much calcium) in a single population?

And the timing suggests it could be an important factor. Both diseases increased when farming practices changed in North America. Grass contains the precursor to vitamin K2 that animals convert for us. When animal feed was changed to grains to simplify production, the animals no longer ate grass and other plants containing chlorophyll, the green substance in plants with the pre-ingredient they needed to produce K2. Without realizing the difference, we dramatically changed the vitamin K2 content of our diet. Not only are you what you eat, you are what your food eats!

Vitamin K1 is found in green leafy vegetables, the broccoli/cauliflower family of vegetables, and small amounts in meat, fish and eggs. Animals and some bacteria can convert K1 into K2, but humans cannot, although our gut bacteria can convert a small amount. To get the recommended amount, we need to consume it regularly in our diet as we don't store this nutrient.

Choosing grass-fed meat and pastured eggs (from hens that feed in a pasture) can correct a vitamin K deficiency. Since beta-carotene (a yellow nutrient) and chlorophyll (the green stuff in plants that animals make into vitamin K) usually occur together, butter and egg yolks that contain vitamin K are darker yellow. When visiting Spain, I've noticed that egg yolks there are a deep golden colour, so I suspect that hens there must be allowed to feed in pastures. Perhaps that's one reason the Spanish are one of the healthiest populations!

Cheese is produced by bacterial action on milk, and some of these bacteria produce vitamin K2 at the same time. So, some cheeses also contain vitamin K2. Some of us also have bacteria in our digestive systems that can convert K1 to K2, but these bacteria can't produce enough K2 to satisfy our needs.

If you can't find grass-fed food or fermented products with the vitamin, you can take a vitamin K2 supplement. K2 is also called menaquinone or MK and, just to make it complicated, there are several varieties of MK, depending on whether they are produced by animals or bacteria. MK-4 comes from animal sources. One source suggests it works well but is cleared from the bloodstream quickly, so requires dosing several times a day. Menaquinone-7 (MK-7) comes from plant sources, and it is suggested to be a better choice as it stays active with once a day dosing. However, both types work to correct a vitamin K2 deficiency, even if one source may be slightly better than the other.

So, I plan to buy my eggs from local farmers when possible in the future and will ask whether they let them out of the coup once in a while. And I'll be looking for a vitamin K2 supplement for the days when I don't have nice yellow-yolked eggs or grass-fed meat! What about you?

If you want to know more, here are two references:

Vitamin K2 and the Calcium Paradox by Kate Rheaume-Bleue, BSc, ND

Vitamin K2—A little known nutrient can make a big difference in heart and bone health https://www.todaysdietitian.com/newarchives/060113p54.shtml

# Chapter 7: Is it Dangerous to Be Overweight?

## The "Weight debate..."

The BMI (Body Mass Index) classes body weight into 4 categories: underweight, normal, overweight and obese. But if you assumed that being "normal" weight was best for your health, you would be wrong, according to statistics...

There are many online calculators available to check your BMI. Most will also tell you which category you fall into. Just search "Body Mass Index" or check out the link I have posted on my website in the references for this book.

Now, let me tell you about a study published in the Journal of the American Medical Association (JAMA) back in 2005... It was entitled "Excess deaths associated with underweight, overweight, and obesity". But in the results section, it states: "Overweight was <u>not</u> associated with excess mortality" (emphasis added).

The study found that being in the overweight group was associated with a significantly <u>reduced</u> mortality... those who were "overweight" had an increased life expectancy. Yes, that's worth repeating... Those who were "overweight" lived the longest - longer than those who were underweight, normal weight or obese (very overweight)[12].

But, most medical information sites (including the one I link to above) continue to state that being overweight is harmful to health... similar to obesity, but not as bad—a sort of "obesity lite", as one author described it.

Another Canadian study, entitled "BMI and Mortality: Results From a National Longitudinal Study of Canadian Adults" published in Obesity journal in 2010[13] divided those in the obese group and found that even the "obesity I" class (but not the heavier "obesity II" class) had lower mortality than the "normal" class of BMI.

So, with this evidence, why do many medical professionals and online websites continue to pressure us to reduce body weight lower than is necessary to reduce risk to health? It is well established that many people, especially women, have issues with body image, with thinness being widely promoted as the ideal we should struggle to achieve. But these studies strongly suggest that we are reducing our life expectancy if we stay too slim.

Physician and author, Malcolm Kendrick, suggests this may be because of an unspoken rule of sorts in medicine: not to question those in authority, not to "buck the system". Family doctors defer to the opinions of specialists and organizations, and success (and hospital privileges!) sometimes bypass those who ask uncomfortable questions.

I've noticed this. When asked for an opinion on the cholesterol controversy (discussed in a previous chapter), my husband's family physician said that GPs simply follow recommendations from the specialists. And when we asked my husband's specialist what he thought about the controversy, he said he hadn't read it and invited us to submit the article I'd read. We dropped off 3 articles to him, with our email clearly written on the front, but received no reply at all! I was surprised—I expected to at least receive some sort of rebuttal and was hoping to get a specialist's opinion about the controversy, something that would help me feel better about my husband taking one of these medications...

Perhaps something similar is happening in the "weight debate"... the BMI calculation is too well established for mere front-line doctors to challenge it. No one wants to go against the "status quo". However, a friend told me that her family doctor advises adding an extra 10 pounds as one ages, as he has observed himself that this additional weight enabled his patients to cope with disease more easily as they aged, with greater chance of surviving a serious illness.

So, is it dangerous to your health to be moderately overweight? Studies suggest that it's not only OK, but it's beneficial to your health to carry a little extra weight as you age! It's time to update BMI charts...

# Plastic: Another contributor to obesity...

A growing body of evidence suggests that plastic is making us gain weight. A common ingredient in plastic, Bisphenol A (BPA), is the suspected culprit...it's a "hormone disruptor" that interferes with the normal actions of our hormones leading to an imbalance that can cause an increase in body weight.

BPA has been identified as an "obesogen"... a chemical that can inappropriately change stability of fat metabolism and storage (or "fat homeostasis"), change setpoints of metabolism, disrupt energy balance or change the regulation of appetite and feeling of satiety (or fullness) to promote fat accumulation and obesity.

A study in 2012 found that children and teenagers who had higher levels of BPA in their urine were more likely to be overweight. Similar results were found in studies of adults. Data from the American Centers for Disease Control (CDC) show that 92.6% of people age 6 and over have detectable levels of BPA in their urine.

Worries about BPA toxicity have led to BPA-free products being produced, using BPS and BPF instead. But are these products safer?

They may not be. A study, published in the Journal of the Endocrine Society in July 2019, suggests that all bisphenols are linked with obesity and weight gain. Although diet and exercise are still considered the major factors in controlling weight, these chemicals may also be a factor.

Researchers point out that an association between bisphenols and obesity doesn't prove they cause weight gain. They say more research is needed. However, this is just another reason to avoid use of plastic, and especially to ensure that it doesn't come in contact with your food and drinks. Transfer of chemicals from plastic to food is more likely to occur when the food is hot or contains fats or oils, since these hormone-disrupting chemicals usually dissolve in fats and oils, just like our own hormones do.

So, choose foods that are sold in paper, cloth or metal containers or, better yet, are sold in bulk with no packaging. Aim to buy drinks that are packaged in glass bottles.

While you're helping to reduce plastic waste and heal the environment, you may also improve your health and your waistline!

*References:*

Definition of "obesogen" (Wikipedia) https://en.wikipedia.org/wiki/Obesogen

Chemical in Plastic Linked to Childhood Obesity https://www.livescience.com/36655-bpa-childhood-obesity-chemical-plastic.html

BPA-Free But Still Dangerous? Replacement Chemicals Linked to Childhood Obesity https://www.livescience.com/66026-bpa-replacement-chemicals-childhood-obesity.html

# Chapter 8: The Environment: Where do Drugs We Swallow Eventually Go?

## The drugs we take don't just "disappear... they are excreted

Researchers at the University of Buffalo have discovered that human antidepressants and their breakdown products are building up in the brains of fish in the Niagara River that flows between Lake Erie and Lake Ontario. Researchers at two universities in Thailand have confirmed these results.

The researchers started out by looking for a variety of chemicals that are in human medications and personal care products. They checked the organs and muscles of 10 species of fish, and antidepressants stood out as the major problem. All 10 species they checked had detectable levels of these drugs.

How is this happening? The drugs they found: Zoloft, Celexa, Prozac and Sarafem (another brand name for Prozac), are widely used in both the US and Canada. Usage increased by 65% between 1999 and 2014, according to the US National Center for Health Statistics. The drugs people take do not magically disappear—they pass out of the body through the urine, feces and/or sweat, sometimes intact and sometimes changed to a slightly different form that may be more or less active than the original drug. Water treatment systems do not remove these drugs, allowing them to flow into lakes and rivers where fish live, along with treated wastewater.

Worse, levels of antidepressants found in fish brains were several times higher than the concentration in the water, suggesting that the drugs are gradually accumulating in fish. When fish are exposed to a drug but cannot break it down or clear it from their bodies, this can cause accumulating amounts to be stored... in this case, in the fish's brains.

The species tested were smallmouth bass, largemouth bass, rudd, rock bass, white bass, white perch, walleye, bowfin, steelhead and yellow perch. The rock bass had the highest concentrations of antidepressants, but several fish had a variety of drugs in their bodies and all 10 species tested were found to have some level of antidepressants.

The good news (if you can call it that...) is that we don't eat fish brains, so this makes it less likely for the drugs to affect humans. But what about the fish? It is not yet known how these drugs might alter their health and behaviour, but other studies suggest they can affect feeding behaviour or survival instincts (not noticing predators as readily).

Especially if your drinking water originally comes from a lake or river, it's possible you're being exposed to a low-level cocktail of drugs. On the positive side, water treatment plants that follow established standards remove 90 to 95% of pharmaceuticals from drinking water, so we are exposed to much lower levels than fish in rivers and lakes. Many experts have felt that the drug levels in drinking water, being much lower than a person would take as treatment, could not have a significant effect. However, no one really knows whether a mixture of many active drugs, consumed at low levels over a lifetime, is a risk to people's health.

A group of researchers found levels high enough to be "of environmental concern" in the Great Lakes and Minnesota River that included traces of acetaminophen (Tylenol), codeine, antibiotics, hormones, steroids, anti-epileptic drugs and dozens of other chemicals.

Health Canada reportedly found traces of drugs in samples of drinking water that came from lakes and rivers across Canada. Their report has not yet been published but was described in an article on cbc.ca website (see reference below).

Some experts particularly worry about effects on the hormone systems and immune system. Researchers have discussed a potential link between hormones from birth control pills that end up in the environment (along with other compounds with estrogen-like activity, such as certain pesticides) and the risk of prostate cancer. Scientists have already proven that these chemicals are creating "intersex" fish—male fish who have developed eggs in their testicles—putting the survival of certain species at risk in some waterways.

Wastewater treatment plants focus on killing disease-causing bacteria and removing solid matter, nitrogen, phosphorus and dissolved organic carbon. However, they pay little or no attention to drugs, hormones and chemicals that might be in human urine. Fish, especially those who live near sewage outlets, are being exposed to a cocktail of drugs 24 hours a day and it is not known whether humans exposed to a low-level mixture of active drugs could be affected too. Its time to look at ways to remove these chemicals from wastewater and prevent their release into the environment. An unhealthy environment will eventually affect our health and that of wildlife.

*References:*

http://www.cbc.ca/news/technology/
human-antidepressants-building-up
[1]-in-brains-of-fish-in-niagara-river-1.4274735[2]

http://www.cbc.ca/news/health/
drinking-water-contaminated-by-excret
[3]ed-drugs-a-growing-concern-1.2772289[4]

---

1. http://www.cbc.ca/news/technology/

   human-antidepressants-building-up-in-brains-of-fish-in-niagara-river-1.4274735

2. http://www.cbc.ca/news/technology/

   human-antidepressants-building-up-in-brains-of-fish-in-niagara-river-1.4274735

3. http://www.cbc.ca/news/health/

   drinking-water-contaminated-by-excreted-drugs-a-growing-concern-1.2772289

4. http://www.cbc.ca/news/health/

   drinking-water-contaminated-by-excreted-drugs-a-growing-concern-1.2772289

First Nations Food, Nutrition & Environment Study (funded by Health Canada) http://www.fnfnes.ca/docs/ FNFNES_Ontario_Regional_Report_2014_final[5].pdf[6]

https://www.health.harvard.edu/newsletter_article/drugs-in-the-water

https://www.pbs.org/wgbh/nova/article/pharmaceuticals-in-the-water/

5. http://www.fnfnes.ca/docs/FNFNES_Ontario_Regional_Report_2014_final.pdf

6. http://www.fnfnes.ca/docs/FNFNES_Ontario_Regional_Report_2014_final.pdf

# Save our Waters, Wetlands and Tourism (SWWAT)

I had a great discussion with my neighbour about issues that increase the risk of pollution on our beaches. Initially concerned about the impact of a large proposed campground nearby, she quickly realized that the greater issue is damage to the delicate ecology of the shoreline along the entire coast of our province. This led her to become involved in a growing movement to protect our New Brunswick, Canada coastline. She established a local group, along with another concerned neighbour, to create awareness in members of our village council about coastal pollution concerns.

They subsequently joined forces with 3 other similar groups in nearby communities, creating a large group that has been named SWWAT (Save our Waters, Wetlands and Tourism) to have a stronger voice with our New Brunswick provincial government. I joined them in attending meetings with others living on the NB coast, from Shediac to Murray Beach. We exchanged ideas and discussed future actions we could take to identify and correct existing problems and to prevent development of future problems along the NB coastline.

The issues are similar along the entire Atlantic coastline in Canada, and the US. Wetlands have been seen as "wasteland" and simply filled in to create developments for human use. Even my home was built into the wetland before existing regulations were in place several years before we bought it. We have returned a swath of land on our property to natural vegetation along an area of water drainage from higher ground, both to restore some filtration function that was lost and because we love the appearance of the natural vegetation.

As I thought about what we had discussed after talking to my neighbours and attending the SWWAT meeting, I wondered what I could do to help. I realized that this is an issue of education and awareness:

- We need to educate people who use the coastline for recreation or work that every small action is cumulative—everyone needs to be aware each action that causes a small amount of damage can add together to cause significant problems for humans, birds, sea life and the overall ecosystem of the coastline.

- We need to create awareness in municipal and provincial government employees and elected politicians who make decisions that affect our shores:
    - about the facts around issues that are causing damage now;
    - about finding and correcting the sources of existing problems that are potential health hazards;
    - and about the importance of considering both the current and future impact of their decisions and legislation.
- It isn't simply about testing water quality so Public Health can predict when beaches should be closed, it's about finding and correcting the causes of bacteria in coastal waters and taking action through legislation and policy that will correct existing problems and prevent future deterio ration of ecological systems along our shores.
- We also need to educate our youth—the next generation—to ensure this wonderful resource is available in the future. Just on our small stretch of beach, we have had late night fires that consumed snow fencing used to prevent erosion of dunes and burned Christmas trees placed against damaged dune areas to encourage rebuilding. We've also had to pick up broken glass and garbage from impromptu midnight beach parties and careless beach bathers! But youth can also be a passionate force for positive change, educating their parents at the same time. We realized that the way to reach young people is through engaging their schools and increasing our reach through social media and our website.
- We need to continue to research solid facts surrounding this issue and communicate these to government and the public to create knowledge and an awareness of the severity of the problem.
- We want to continue to engage the attention of news media to enable wider awareness of coastline concerns.

Because I am a blogger and had already created a website and marketing materials for my pharmacy business, I volunteered to work on similar approaches to help spread the word about these environmental issues. It's not only the health of those like me who use the beaches for recreation, but also the tourism, fisheries and ultimately the economic health of coastal areas that are at stake.

The group's goal is to create legislation to foster long-term protection and reduction in development of coastlines and waterways. This will protect the health and safety of families and visitors to the beaches, and the future of the tourism and fisheries industries in the area.

Will you join the cause to protect waterways and coastlines? How healthy are the shores, lakes and rivers in your area? These issues are of concern in all waterways, oceans, lakes and rivers, not just those in coastal New Brunswick.

# How can we make change easier?

The metric system, smoking, carbon tax and reducing plastic pollution all require us to accept change to make things better in the future... for our children and our grandchildren. What can we do to make change easier when it's really important?

**The Metric System**

Canada changed from miles, ounces and Fahrenheit degrees to the metric system of kilometers, grams and Celsius degrees back in the 1970s. I was in university then and found it easier since my high school science labs had been in metric, but they made it easier by giving measurements, like weather temperatures, food packages and speed signs, in both systems for years until everyone got used to the new system.

We also bought thermometers and rulers with both scales on them. I told my pharmacy customers not to convert fever temperatures but to just remember that 37C was normal and 40C was very high (equal to 104F). For pharmacy students it was a relief...as we had to learn the Canadian system of weights and measures (the same as the British), the American system (with its slightly different ounce and gallon), the metric system AND the obscure Apothecary system with its grains, scruples, drams and ounces (yes... pharmacists have scruples!). It is a relief to use the simple conversions of the metric system!

So, our government legislated this change to bring our systems more in line with the rest of the world, but continued the old system until everyone became used to the alternative ways of measuring.

## Smoking

To discourage smoking, based on research showing second-hand smoking is harmful, cities banned smoking in public and eventually in restaurants and other public areas. This made smoking an activity that could only happen in a special area and was no longer acceptable everywhere as it had been. Along with government-sponsored education, this "de-normalization" of smoking has led to steadily decreasing rates of smoking in North America.

A combination of restricting where smoking was acceptable and educating people why it was dangerous worked to change behaviour gradually. However, I read that smoking rates have increased again recently, possibly because of the availability and popularity of e-cigarettes. There's still more work for governments to do to eliminate this harmful habit, but there are fewer cigarette smokers now than there once were!

And a note about e-cigarettes... the chemicals used in these devices have never been tested for long-term use by inhalation. Reports suggest that heavy use of e-cigarettes may be associated with an unusual lung disease not seen before.

## Carbon Tax

The Carbon Tax is a fee imposed on polluting carbon-based fuels, like coal, oil and gas. While the tax is much debated, experts say it will change behaviour: The tax will encourage people to choose products and services that are less polluting to avoid the tax. Nothing like money to make people consider changing! Our Canadian government tells us our version of this tax will be revenue-neutral for government and much of the population - the tax collected will be rebated to consumers—but studies say it will still work as an incentive to change.

## Plastics

There's an enormous problem with plastic that most of us don't see... tons of plastic waste are ending up in our oceans and lakes, and it takes many years to degrade. As it breaks down, it becomes "microplastic" that enters our food supply. Substances in plastics affect our hormone function and our health.

So, what can be learned from other system changes we've made that we can apply to plastics? We need awareness, education, and system changes to make us want to correct what we're doing. Scientists estimate that by 2050 there will be more plastic by weight in oceans than sea life... it's time to change.

**Here are 9 suggestions for things you can do:**

1.  Use reusable items instead of disposable:
    a.  This includes bags, cutlery, straws, coffee cups, plastic wrap and anything else you can think of.
2.  Stop buying bottled water.
    a.  Filter water instead and use reusable bottles. You can even get bottles with a filter built in!
3.  Boycott products with plastic microbeads, such as soaps, body wash, toothpaste.
    a.  These tiny beads often slip through water treatment systems and look like food to fish.
    b.  Microbeads are already banned in some countries.
4.  Cook more at home to avoid packaging.
    a.  If you order out for dining at home, ask that no cutlery be added to your order.
5.  Buy second-hand.
    a.  Second-hand items are not packaged, you'll prevent these items from ending up in a landfill and you'll save money!
6.  Recycle
    a.  Already many communities require us to separate plastics and other items in our garbage, so they can be recycled. And

in some communities, if you don't, they may just leave your garbage at the curb (my friends call them the garbage police!). So changes are happening at the community level. However, not all communities take part in separating and recycling garbage. If yours doesn't, suggest it!

    b.   And recycle in your home too! Reusing plastic bags and containers means fewer will end up in the garbage.

7.  Support bag charges and bans.

    a.   These can be one of the fastest ways to make people change their habits quickly and our local government has banned most single-use plastics, like straws and grocery bags.

    b.   Get a few small reusable bags that you can carry in your purse or keep a few in the back seat of the car and remember to take them with you into the store. I do both of these!

8.  Buy in bulk (yogurt, snacks, etc.).

    a.   Buy large sizes and repackage these into reusable containers, or better yet, make your own snacks! They might be tastier and better for you too...

9.  Put pressure on manufacturers and retailers to change.

    a.   Email, Tweet, or just buy elsewhere when you notice bad plastic practices!

Please watch the short video on the plastic problem on the Plastic Pollution Coalition website (see link below)[14] Besides further explaining the problems we are facing with excess use of single-use plastic, there are links to information on how to reduce the problem and live "plastic free".

# Chapter 9: What Activities Can Help Us Live Healthier and Longer?

## Family dinners are good for your health!

I remember Sunday dinners that seemed to go on for hours when I was growing up. My grandparents would join us, we'd have dinner, then coffee for the adults, and just hang around the table talking for ages. My dad loved to get an animated discussion going, often about current news or about mischief he and his brother did as kids (that was our favourite topic!).

So, it struck a chord when I read about a study done in Quebec that conducted surveys of families with young children to find out whether the environment during a typical family meal might influence learning, lifestyle and socializing.

They began by surveying families with 6-year-olds to determine the environment of a typical family meal. Four years later, when the children were age 10, they conducted more surveys: asking parents to assess their children's lifestyle habits, teachers to gauge academic achievement, and the children themselves to assess their social adjustment from their point of view.

They found that improved family meal environment quality (eating together and engaging in conversation during the meal), predicted higher levels of physical fitness, decreased soft drink consumption, and reduced physical aggression, oppositional behaviour, delinquency and reactive aggression.

Survey reports tell us the frequency of family meals is in decline. The Euromonitor International's annual study of global consumers shows a world-wide trend towards less structured meal occasions, resulting from busy lifestyles, more unconventional working hours, increased single-parent households and increased numbers of working women.

Breakfast, once a regular sit-down meal, has become less consistent and we often now eat it on the run or skip it altogether. Snacking has increased because of smaller breakfasts and shorter lunch breaks (with many eating in their car while doing errands or even at their desks due to work pressures), leading to an increased demand for pre-packaged portable foods, unfortunately often highly preserved to increase shelf-life.

The annual study found that younger, urban consumer groups have been trending towards more flexible and informal eating habits. Only approximately half still cook a meal entirely from raw ingredients at least once a week.

However, Quebec researchers also found a recent trend toward eating in rather than out and, when eating out, frequenting less expensive locations. They reported that the trend in recent years toward eating more at home was likely because of financial pressures from the recession that began in 2008, and with the current pandemic, this trend is increasing. Use of prepared ingredients, such as sauces, is also on the rise, making home-cooked meals easier to prepare. The researchers' opinion was that now would be a good time for a public awareness program to encourage more frequent family dinners with conversation between adults and children—what they termed a quality eating environment.

Many of us only enjoy family dinners on special holidays. The studies described above suggest that we should make these a regular event, especially if there are small children in the family.

But socialization is important for adults, too. Studies of communities around the world with higher proportions of centenarians (people over 100 years old), referred to by researchers as "Blue Zones", looked for shared characteristics. This is a list of what these communities had in common:

- Family and social engagement
- Semi-vegetarianism (majority of food from plant sources)
- Legumes commonly consumed
- Consistent moderate physical activity as part of life
- Less smoking

This list seems to fit with eating food at home in a family environment. Quality family time improves physical, academic and social outcomes for young children that persist for years. It also echoes Michael Pollan's food rules ("Eat real food, mostly plants, and not too much") that I discussed in one of my blogs.

Having a longer and healthier life does not have to be complicated. Planning simple meals that include plenty of fruits and vegetables, eating with family and friends when possible, and keeping active throughout the day to stay fit are good places to start. Some claim you could add 10 quality years to your life by following this simple strategy.

Now, doesn't that sound like a good plan?

# What Can I Do to Improve Sleep Problems?

Ideal sleep for an average adult means falling asleep within 30 minutes, not waking more than once, and taking less than 20 minutes to return to sleep when you do wake at night. Is your sleep less than ideal? If so, this chapter is for you!

Here are some tips to help get the rest you need:

1. **Turn off electronics**. Phones, tablets and computers bleep and flash and these noises can disturb your sleep. Don't charge your electronics in your bedroom or set them to "do not disturb" during the night. If you like to read your devices before bed, check if there is a "blue light filter" you can turn on. Blue light is more stimulating than other types and is more likely to keep you awake.
2. **Daytime naps?** While brief naps can recharge and improve productivity, longer ones can leave you groggy and make it more difficult to get a good night's sleep. Limit daytime naps to 20 minutes or fewer.
3. **Watching the clock?** Some find they check the time frequently when they wake at night, getting upset about being unable to get back to sleep quickly. If this is you, turning the clock away from view or putting it in a drawer can mean a better night's sleep.
4. **Get comfy...** A relaxing bath with Epsom salts can relieve muscle and joint pains and set you up for a good rest. If your bed is not comfortable, consider a new mattress or memory foam topper. Your pillow needs to be the right depth to support the natural curve of your neck, and a second pillow for between or under your knees may make you more comfortable, especially if you have issues with back pain. A dark, relatively cool room also helps sleep.
5. **Allergies?** If you get stuffy at night, you may be allergic to dust mites, one of the most common allergies. These are microscopic creatures that live off dead skin cells in our mattresses and pillows. Dust mite proof or plastic mattress covers that are wiped down or vacuumed regularly plus washing bedding (including pillows) in hot water

reduces mite counts and can eliminate or reduce this problem. Replace any old pillows, as these often have high counts of dust and dust mites.

6. **Stick to sleep and sex**... Working, watching TV or surfing the internet in bed trains your brain to be alert in the bedroom. Make your sleep environment a relaxing one by saving it for only sleep and sex.

7. **Wake/sleep cycle...** Establish routine bed and wake times. This can help people of any age fall asleep more quickly and sleep more soundly. Lowering lights in the evening also helps set you up for sleep and bright light for 5 to 30 minutes when you wake up helps get you going in the morning too.

8. **Avoid caffeine**. Some people who don't metabolize caffeine well may find that any caffeine results in a poor night's sleep. For most, avoiding caffeine after noontime is usually sufficient. Watch for hidden caffeine in chocolate and some "herbal" teas, pain relievers, and weight loss pills.

9. **Exercise** can help or hinder. Regular exercise can improve sleep, but some experience a post-workout increase in energy that could keep you awake. Try scheduling exercise to finish 3 to 4 hours before bedtime. Relaxing exercise, like yoga or tai chi, however, can help sleep when done just before bed.

10. **Alcohol**. Booze can make you drowsy but, when the effect wears off, you may wake up more often. Mid-life women may actually experience increased hormone swings several hours after consuming alcohol. Try non-caffeine herbal tea instead if you notice this connection.

11. **Getting up to pee?** Try avoiding liquids for 2 hours before bed.

12. **Noises at night?** Use earplugs or try a white noise machine or fan to drown out traffic, a dripping faucet, hubby's snoring or the neighbour's barking dog.

13. **Still smoking?** Nicotine is a stimulant that can make insomnia worse... yet another good reason to quit!

14. **And doggie makes three...** You love your pet, but he can cause nighttime wakening and allergies. Ask your vet or pet school how to

train your pet to sleep in his own bed. Same goes for toddlers—but talk to a sleep specialist or your doctor instead of the vet...

15. **Consider meditation.** Meditation trains you to put active thoughts out of your mind. Clearing your thoughts for even 10 mins before bed can help you fall asleep. Avoiding work or complex discussions for 2 to 3 hours before you retire is also advised for best sleep. My hubby is great at this—he tells me he simply makes his mind go blank and regularly falls asleep in about two minutes!

16. **Careful with sleeping pills**. Many prescription sleeping medications are habit forming and only recommended for up to 7 days of continuous use. Rebound insomnia can occur with guaranteed poor sleep for up to several weeks on discontinuation. Some also have side effects such as memory impairment, and use in the elderly is associated with falls that can cause bone fractures. Slowly tapering down the dose before stopping can help reduce rebound insomnia.

17. **Non-prescription supplements?**
    a. A **magnesium** supplement taken at bedtime relaxes muscles and can help sleep. Magnesium is important for bone health too, so you may benefit from it in multiple ways... and it's better absorbed on an empty stomach.
    b. **Chamomile** or **valerian** in pill or tea form can help sleep and are non-addicting. Valerian smells somewhat like "dirty socks", though, so I'd suggest the pill form of it!
    c. **Vitamin B5 (pantothenic acid)** can help reduce production of the stress hormone, cortisol, that we sometimes produce inappropriately at nighttime when stressed, causing us to wake at night feeling "tired but wired". B5 is a common ingredient in vitamin B-based stress formulas available without prescription. And it's just as effective if taken in a standard B-Complex formula.
    d. **Antihistamines**, like Gravol (dimenhydrinate) or Benadryl (diphenhydramine, also used in several non-prescription sleep aids), are not recommended for nightly use. Both have been reported to be habit forming and tolerance develops to the drowsy effect within a few days, leading some to increase

the dose inappropriately. Regular users may notice withdrawal effects when stopping the drug.

18. **Look for a potential cause.** Ask your doctor if the cause of the problem could be a health condition like acid reflux, arthritis, asthma, depression or hormone imbalance. Get your pharmacist to check if a medication you are taking could contribute to insomnia. Try keeping a sleep diary to determine what factors might interfere with your sleep. Ask about the possibility of treatment at a sleep clinic.

Lastly, until you find the solution to your problem, avoid tossing and turning in bed. Get up and do something calming, like reading or just looking out the window for a few minutes. Chances are you'll fall asleep more easily when you return to bed!

# Chapter 10: How Can I Improve My Memory?

## Make a note...

My mom had the best memory of anyone in the family. She always kept notes... about everyday things: the weather, appointments, who visited, prices of things, interesting articles in the news.

And now there's research that says we remember better when we write something down and recall more when using pen and paper than when we type on a computer.

Researchers have found that physical writing uses more parts of the brain than typing does and involving multiple senses helps us remember better. Years ago, I learned we remember more when we both hear and see information compared to just reading it. And doing something (anything!) with the information, whether using it or simply playing a game with the information, helps us remember even more—all because we're using more of our senses.

All this suggests that children should learn to write, not just use a keyboard. The slower speed of writing and the increased difficulty of altering what you've already put down makes you organize your thoughts more concisely. As an adult, if you're reading an important book or information article, take notes. Writing down what's important to you will help you remember the details and organize the information in your mind.

There's something about pens and paper I've always loved... a special pen, multiple colours of ink, a beautiful hardcover notebook to write in. Perhaps that's part of why I like to write. So, perhaps I'll start a journal—one on paper. I tried an online version a few years ago, which offered the bonus of allowing you to add photos, but it seems what I wrote just disappeared into a list of dates. And maybe I'll look for a really nice pen to write it with...

How about you? Want to improve your memory? Try making notes of what you want to remember, or things you'd like to accomplish. Review your notes later to help your recall of the facts and check off items on your "to do" list—you may find that you feel better about your memory and your achievements!

# Mid-life Memory Problems

Have you ever gone to the kitchen or bedroom, then forgotten what you wanted to do there once you'd arrived? Have you ever been unable to find a common word or lost your train of thought, mid-conversation? It's enough to make you worry you might be losing your mind... and it happens to too many of us after age 50 or even 40...

Yes, it's happened to me too—so embarrassing and frustrating—and to many of my friends and family. We try to laugh it off as an "old-timer moment" or a "brain fart" although secretly we worry it might be an early sign of serious memory problems. But how would you know? I did some reading to see what I could learn...

Like every part of the body, your brain cells age over the years. Researchers once thought we were born with all the brain cells we would ever have, but in more recent years they've realized this isn't correct. Your brain is "plastic"—it grows and changes with use, creating new nerve cell branches and connections as you add memories and learn new skills. And new neurons are created too, a process called "neurogenesis".

**"Use it or lose it"**

So, the first piece of advice for maintaining an excellent memory, is to continue to learn throughout your life so you will constantly create new brain nerve cells (called neurons) and new connections between these neurons in your brain. If you aren't building new connections and reinforcing old ones by using them, the number of connections (and the efficiency of your brain!) will gradually decrease. And it's never too late to start...

The more complex the skill is that you are learning and the less familiar you are with the concept, the better it is for your brain function. For example, learning a new language is highly recommended to keep your overall brain function sharp. I guess I made an excellent decision when I started learning Spanish a few years ago. Trying something that is out of your comfort zone is also recommended, as you will need to work harder at learning—presumably creating more new brain pathways in the effort.

Another approach you could consider, to use and build your brain, is one of the online "brain exercise" games. One I came across, MyBrainTrainer.com,[15] is worth looking at, especially if you have frequent memory problems and want a simple way to exercise your memory. It uses a gaming format and compares your scores with their average user, so you can track your improvement. It's free for the first 3 months to see if you find it useful.

**Diet**

The second piece of advice I learned is to look at your diet. While a healthy, balanced diet is recommended to support all parts of the body, fats are needed for healthy brain cells, and specifically omega-3 fats. Nerve cells in the brain have a fatty coating called myelin, that you could think of as "insulation". When it becomes damaged, the nerve can short-circuit. In Multiple Sclerosis, many nerves lose their myelin protection, and nerve signals to muscles and organs (such as the eyes) can completely fail, resulting in inability to move or blindness. In the brain, with its billions of nerve cells, losing the function of individual neurons is not always so obvious.

Seafood is an excellent source of omega-3 fats but be aware that some fish contain methyl mercury which can harm your memory, especially large fish like tuna (albacore and ahi tuna), swordfish and shark. They eat smaller fish, concentrating any mercury they contain. Fish caught in lakes that contain large amounts of run-off surface water (the Great Lakes, for example) can also contain increased amounts of mercury. Salmon, shrimp, tilapia, canned light tuna and catfish are believed to have lower mercury levels, on average. And little fish like sardines, anchovies, and scallops are also less likely to contain the chemical, being lower in the food chain that concentrates mercury.

An omega-3 supplement that has been tested for methyl mercury content might be a good choice to increase your intake, unless you can verify the mercury content of the seafood you purchase. If you don't like seafood, or have an allergy to it, MCT (medium chain triglycerides) oil is an alternative "good fat" that can be taken as a supplement. Other food sources of omega-3 fats include flax seeds, chia seeds, Brussels sprouts, hemp seeds, and walnuts.

The primary fuel for your brain is glucose, so eating complex carbohydrates is thought to be helpful for memory. These foods—such as whole grains, beans, peas and vegetables—release their glucose more slowly, keeping your brain supplied with its favourite fuel much longer than simple sugary foods do.

You also want to avoid "brain rust" — oxidation damage to your brain cells. Oxidation is a natural process: oxygen radicals, produced as a by-product of our metabolism, cause damage to healthy cells. Although debated, the theory says that as we age, we become less efficient at repairing the damage oxygen radicals cause. Eating antioxidant foods helps prevent as much damage from occurring by neutralizing these oxidation by-products. Colourful fruits and vegetables contain lots of antioxidants, hence the recommendation to serve a colourful plate. But other foods can contain high levels of antioxidants too. These include onions, artichokes and potatoes; green and black tea; red wine, grape juice, and pomegranate juice; nuts, such as peanuts with their skin, almonds and pecans; and spices, such as cinnamon and turmeric. It's been reported that in India, where the average diet contains plenty of turmeric-containing curry and seafood, the occurrence of Alzheimer's disease is one-quarter of the rate in North America. There may be a connection...

References:

Carved in Sand—Cathryn Jakobson Ramin

Mercury guide https://www.nrdc.org/stories/mercury-guide

Progesterone: The Multiple Roles of a Remarkable Hormone—Dr. John Lee

Healthline - https://www.healthline.com/nutrition/7-plant-sources-of-omega-3sTOC_TITLE_HDR_2

There are many factors that can dull your memory... Here are a few more to be aware of:

## Sleep

Getting a good night's sleep is crucial to having your brain perform at its best. However, sleeping pills can leave you drowsy and can even impair your memory. There are many ways to improve your sleep, starting with good "sleep hygiene" or sleep habits. A good place to start is reading the Sleep Well Nova Scotia website[16], created by the Nova Scotia government to help reduce use of sleep pills.

## Hormones: Estrogen and Progesterone

Hormones can help to improve brain function. Sufficient levels of estrogen and progesterone are necessary for optimal function of the centers for memory and decision-making (the frontal lobe and hippocampus of the brain), and to increase neurogenesis (formation of new nerve cells). We also need these hormones to properly use the neurotransmitter, acetylcholine, that passes messages from one neuron to the next.

Estrogen acts as an antioxidant and appears to reduce the effects of beta-amyloid (the protein that researchers suspect causes problems in Alzheimer's Disease). Studies of women who take estrogen supplements after menopause report improved brain function, but those who take the synthetic progestin, medroxyprogesterone, along with it, do not. Unfortunately, real progesterone has not been tested widely for its effects on the brain. However, researchers have identified progesterone receptors on the myelin that protects nerves, showing that it is active in this tissue.

I recall a co-worker who had early menopause explaining the difference she noticed in herself when she changed from medroxyprogesterone, which was causing several side effects, to progesterone capsules. She had been having difficulty remembering drug names (so embarrassing for a pharmacist!) but improved dramatically after the drug switch to having no difficulty with names at all. I also had several women clients who referred to their progesterone cream (that I compounded for them) as their "memory cream", as they had noticed a difference with its use. I suspect it would only have this effect if the woman was lacking progesterone, but this is an area where we need more research.

However, research into hormone effects on the brain (and elsewhere) slowed after the release of the results of the Women's Health Initiative (WHI) study in 2002. Although the goal of this study was to examine the benefits of estrogen in older women who were well past menopause (the date of their last period), the results were thought to apply to all women, and many doctors and patients thought the hormones were too dangerous for general use.

Reanalysis of the results of the WHI study and further studies have shown that hormone replacement provides more benefit than risk if started soon after menopause to control symptoms of hormonal change. Doctors are prescribing hormones more frequently again when women have significant complaints of hormone imbalance or lack of hormones. Women at risk of breast cancer, blood clots, or heart disease, however, are still recommended to avoid use, and doctors screen women carefully before prescribing hormones. Now, hormones that are exactly the same as those produced by women's bodies are available in tablets, creams and patches, and these seem to be a better choice. It is recommended to use the lowest amount of any hormone for the shortest time necessary, though, until further long-term safety studies are done. Studies are important to show how long it would be safe to use hormones, especially for issues such as memory and decision-making problems. However, progesterone (the hormone that is the same as the one our bodies make, and that women produce in high amounts during pregnancy) is considered a very safe hormone. Federal law in the US does not require a prescription for its sale, although some pharmacy state laws override this. In Canada, all forms of progesterone require a prescription. The cream form is not commercially available in Canada but can be made by any pharmacist who knows that the base must not contain oil, especially mineral oil, as it blocks absorption of progesterone.

**Cortisol**

Cortisol is a long-acting stress hormone. When it prepares you to deal with a stressful event, it increases blood pressure, speeds the heart, raises cholesterol, and shunts blood away from digestion and toward the muscles to ready them for action. Just this much description of its effects suggests it causes several health problems if it stays in your blood stream constantly because of ongoing stress. Although it is necessary for life and initially sharpens memory and brain functions, too much in your system for too long creates many health problems, including lack of sleep which will dull your memory. Studies in rats showed that excess cortisol caused neurons in the hippocampus (an important area of the brain for memory) to shrink, and reduced branching, connections and formation of new brain nerve cells.

Exposure to stress as a very young child, often results in an increased stress response as an adult. Studies have identified that highly stress-prone adults have considerably more memory impairment and risk of developing Alzheimer's than their non-stressed counterparts. So, not all factors are under our current control for ourselves, although we may be able to make a difference for our children.

But it makes sense to work to reduce stress (and consequently the stress hormones that accompany it), by using techniques like yoga or meditation, as part of a strategy to help improve your memory. Personally, I'm a big fan of just listening to relaxing music or taking a walk on the beach to release stress. But note that vitamin B5 (pantothenic acid) is reported to reduce cortisol levels. Taking this vitamin (or a B-complex vitamin that contains it) at bedtime can help some people with high cortisol get a better night's sleep. Remember that cortisol keeps you awake, activating your stress "fight or flight" system that keeps you alert and ready to fight off danger or run away from it.

**Brain Derived Neurotropic Factor (BDNF)**

Scientists have suggested that cortisol may interfere with the production of Brain Derived Neurotropic Factor (BDNF) which stimulates branching and growth of new brain nerve cells. BDNF is controlled by a particular gene. One-third of humans inherit a variation of this gene that results in poor production of BDNF. So, if you seem to have inherited your mothers "poor memory", maybe you've inherited the less-effective version of this gene. While this is interesting, environmental causes of poor memory are at least as important as the genes you inherited.

On the upside, essential fatty acids, like omega-3's can help to counteract cortisol's effect of reducing growth of new neurons... another reason to have a healthy diet with plenty of "good fats".

**Medications**

We know that sleeping pills and tranquillizers can decrease memory and even cause periods of amnesia in some people. While this may be because of the drowsiness they cause, slowing brain function, it could also be because of the receptors they block in the brain.

Receptor blocking is thought to be the problem with anticholinergic drugs that can cause marked memory decrease in some people. These drugs block the neurotransmitter, acetylcholine, from doing its work in the hippocampus memory center, either as their mode of action or as a side effect. Anti-nausea drugs, antihistamines and some anti-depressants have this anticholinergic effect; the more drowsiness and dry mouth the drug causes as side effects, the greater the anticholinergic effect it has.

Beta-blockers, a class of drugs used for blood pressure and after a heart attack, can also reduce memory, as can some stomach drugs, such as Zantac (ranitidine) and Pepcid (famotidine).

Corticosteroids such as prednisone, which mimic our cortisol, can decrease memory by the same mechanism that high natural cortisol levels can, as described above.

And chemotherapy can cause a general brain fogginess, because of its toxicity, that some patients have nicknamed "chemo brain".

**Diseases and medical conditions**

Lastly, some medical conditions can reduce brain function. Weight loss, where sugar intake is reduced, results in a decreased supply of the brain's favourite food.

Insulin resistance is a condition where the body becomes insensitive to insulin, requiring higher amounts to be released into the blood to move blood sugar into muscle and storage sites. It is present in people with Type 2 diabetes (adult onset) and pre-diabetes. Researchers have found a strong association between people with insulin resistance, those with declining memory, and risk of developing Alzheimer's disease.

Lyme Disease, caused by a bacterium that is carried by infected ticks, can eventually affect brain function and memory if the initial infection is not detected and treated.

Stroke can also affect the memory if it occurs in an area of the brain where memories are processed. And, of course, a brain tumour in one of these areas could show up initially as a memory problem.

So, as with any serious change in your health, it is always wise to consult your doctor if you detect a noticeable change in your memory to find out whether there is a treatable underlying cause of your memory problem.

**Brain "overload"**

One factor that is problematic for our generation is the level of information and distraction we are exposed to daily. Advertisements compete for our attention constantly—advertisers are expert at stealing our focus from what it is we want to accomplish.

We know that to remember something, we need to pay attention, take the information in, process it and store it properly. Studies have shown that multitasking, doing two or more things at once, takes longer than doing each separately. The brain can only focus on one thing at a time and switching between tasks wastes time as we refocus on the alternate activity.

At least some large companies that have been so successful at grabbing our attention now realize the damage they are doing and have talked about changing their strategies. One has even recently rolled out a program recently to meter time on their platform to enable us to regain some control.[17] That might help.

So, if you want to remember something, turn off the social media and its advertising, give what you are doing your full attention and only take on one task at a time.

**Minimal Traumatic Brain Injury**

Next, we know concussions cause brain damage, but minimally traumatic brain injuries can cause problems too, especially if repeated. These are bumps or sudden direction changes that don't cause loss of conscience but are still traumatic enough to create microscopic tears and bleeding in the brain. Sometimes the results only show as headaches or dizziness but can return in mid-life, as memory loss.

# How can you know if it's more than just "age"?

Doctors can use a simple test, called the Mini Mental State Exam (MMSE) to evaluate brain function. It comprises 30 questions that assess language, orientation, calculation, attention, recall and visual-spatial function (the ability to analyze space and visual forms). However, the test is geared to detect people with overt dementia. It isn't sensitive enough to detect early stages of a dementia like Alzheimer's. A person with high mental functioning can drop to normal—a serious change for them—but still test out as having nothing wrong, especially when the various test results are totaled and averaged.

Specialized centers, however, can conduct in-depth memory and brain function tests that detect changes in individual areas of the brain by testing the memory and cognitive functions specific to each area of the brain. These tests are expensive and time-consuming, however, and are not commonly done.

But you don't need to worry if you've just misplaced your keys or lose your train of thought occasionally. However, being unable to find your way home when doing errands, for example, is likely to suggest a more serious problem. But, if you notice a dramatic change in your memory or ability to accomplish daily tasks, it's reason to have a discussion with your doctor.

I hope this chapter has given you some ideas for changes you could make to improve your memory or perhaps has helped you detect an underlying cause of your forgetfulness!

References:

Finding it hard to focus? New York Times https://www.nytimes.com/2018/08/14/style/how-can-i-focus-better.html?rref=collection%2Fsectioncollection%2Fsmarter-livi

Insulin Resistance May Boost Risk of Memory Loss https://www.futurity.org/obesity-memory-alzheimers-insulin-968272/

# Chapter 11: How Can I Reduce My Risk of Stress, Anxiety and Depression?

## Start a Happiness Project

Think of happiness as something you can decide on, something you can practice and get better at... Does that sound strange? Scientists say, the more you choose to focus on being happy and having positive thoughts, the happier you can become.

Your brain is "plastic", as I mentioned earlier. It constantly changes, making new connections as you learn something new or create a fresh memory, and it strengthens the connections that are used most often. Think of a new skill you're learning. The more you practice it, the easier it becomes and the longer you will remember how to do it.

It's the same, experts say, with your thoughts. The more attention you give to the pleasant things in your life, the better you will remember them. Your entire life will just feel happier, because that's what sticks with you.

Darwin's theory, "survival of the fittest", explains how species evolve. Psychologists use the term "Neural Darwinism", or survival of the busiest connections, to refer to our brain's ability to change over time according to what we focus on and learn. Just like muscle, the brain builds up the parts that we use most. Scientists have actually measured thickening in certain parts of the brain that are used more. For example, taxi drivers who memorize streets in large cities have thickened layers in the hippocampus area of their brains, the area where visual-spatial memory, memory for space and visual forms, is stored.

And brain pathways we don't use gradually become weakened and wither. Limiting the time spent dwelling on sad events from the past, for example, means that over time our tendency to pop these thoughts into our mind will lessen. Of course, we all have negative, unpleasant things that happen to us. But if you deal with them as best you can, then set them aside in your thoughts, they will have less impact on your life. This can make you a happier person.

You can also try to find something positive in an unpleasant situation—did you learn something from what happened? Can you do it better next time? Did it bring you closer to those you love? Take any positivity you can and move on. You can't change the past. But you can limit how much effect it has on your future.

For some people, writing a journal of positive thoughts once a day can prompt them to focus on the positive in their lives. For others, simply taking a few seconds to appreciate what is pleasant as it occurs is all they need to do to reinforce these memories and feelings.

So, train your brain to be happy. What you focus on and practice regularly will eventually become an automatic habit. Make it a project to decide consciously every day to dwell on the best things in your life, and likely you will soon find you are a happier person.

Further reading:

The Happiness Habit https://medium.com/thrive-global/the-happiness-habit-7f8f9fef404f

Hardwiring Happiness, by Rick Hanson, PhD

# Stressed? Try using the Relaxation Response

The Relaxation Response essentially functions as the opposite of the Stress Response. Stress increases your heart rate, and blood pressure—which increase risk of heart disease and stroke—as well as your breathing rate and rate of body metabolism. The Relaxation Response does the opposite and has been proposed as a method of reducing the physical effects of stress and decreasing anxiety.

These are the 4 steps to induce the Relaxation Response:

1. Find a quiet environment—decrease outside distractions.
2. Focus on something—repeat a word or sound aloud or in your head, look at a symbol or just down at the ground, or concentrate on a particular feeling (love, happiness) to help eliminate outside thoughts.
3. Keep a passive attitude—empty thoughts from your mind. Do not be concerned about how you are doing.
4. Sit in a comfortable position—you need to remain still for 10—20 minutes. You do not want to fall asleep. Note that these 4 elements will also aid in falling asleep if you are lying down.

It is recommended to practice this relaxation exercise for 10 to 20 minutes, twice a day. Some find the timing in relation to their day's events can make a difference in their results—for example, inducing a relaxation response before bedtime can make it easier to fall asleep.

Many cultures and religious practices, even back in ancient times, include similar forms of exercise as a path to enlightenment, improvement in mood and happiness. The focus can be prayer for those who practice religion—the result is the same: slowed breathing, heart rate, and metabolism; reduced blood pressure; and improved mood. Yoga and transcendental meditation are two examples of cultural practices that are still practiced widely today.

In the distant past, the ability to respond to physical dangers was life saving... the "fight or flight" response that increased blood flow to limbs, increased heart rate and breathing, and increased blood pressure, set humans up to fight off a wild animal or escape from it.

But modern life exposes us to many unique sources of stress, few of which require a physical strength response. Changes in work, family or environment—especially rapid changes—require us to adjust constantly, triggering the same release of stress hormones. Loss of a loved one, especially a spouse, creates high levels of stress and even joyful events, like a promotion, marriage, or a new baby, induce a stress response. Simply living in the city versus a rural area is associated with higher stress, and uncertainty (think of world politics and diseases!) adds to stress too.

Studies have shown that repeated transient surges of stress hormones eventually lead to a permanent increase in blood pressure, also known as "hypertension". This plausibly explains the 90-95% of hypertension of unexplained cause, termed "essential hypertension". Since increased blood pressure is associated with increased risk of heart disease and stroke, practicing the Relaxation Response at least during times of increased stress may be a means to reduce the risk of these diseases. While relaxation exercises are not a substitute for medication in moderate-to-severe hypertension, studies suggest they could add to the effect of medication, allowing lowered doses for control. Studies also suggest practicing the Relaxation Response could avoid development of the condition and could be beneficial in controlling mild forms, along with other lifestyle changes.

However, few doctors ask about your levels of stress at a check up. Stress hormones naturally fluctuate widely during the day, usually being higher in the morning, peaking at each meal, and dropping lower at night. Having low levels at night is a good thing, as the effects of stress hormones keep you alert and awake, and ready for "fight or flight"—not what you want at bedtime! It seems likely that middle of the night awakening, where you're tired but find your mind is racing (described as "tired but wired") may be caused by an inappropriate surge in production of stress hormones in the middle of the night.

Stress is most often treated within the realm of psychology and mental illness, with tranquilizers and antidepressants being prescribed when stress-induced anxiety becomes unbearable. However, learning to trigger the Relaxation Response to reduce the negative effects of stress is side effect-free and costs nothing to practice.

While family physicians receive little formal training in meditation and relaxation techniques, many alternative medicine practitioners use these as part of their therapy. Integration of standard medical treatment and alternative medicine practices like these could result in better treatment for patients and minimization of medications, while reducing cost and decreasing the risk of negative side effects.

This relaxation technique is simple to learn—just follow the 4 steps above. Entering a full relaxation response with lowered blood pressure will become easier and more complete with practice and can make a significant improvement in your health!

Reference: <u>The Relaxation Response</u>, by Herbert Benson MD

# Contributing factors to depression - Robert Sapolsky, Stanford University

Robert Sapolsky is a professor of neuroscience at Stanford University. He researches and teaches students about depression, its causes, and its treatments.

He explains depression as resulting from two types of input: a change in brain transmitters, which we try to correct with antidepressant medications, and thought input, which creates natural release of neurotransmitters and connections between brain neurons, as described earlier.

I liked Sapolsky's description of depression. He explains that healthy normal humans all experience periods of sadness and depression. It's a normal response to traumatic life events. But a normal depression response is limited, and the person gradually recovers within a reasonable time. Depression becomes a problem when the dark mood lingers too long, and the person becomes "stuck" in depression. This is when treatment needs to be considered. Treatments can include both medications and non-medical treatments — both are effective. Non-medical treatments can take more time to exert their effect, but the effect lasts longer after the treatment is stopped. Non-medical treatments also have no side effects or withdrawal effects, both of which are possible with antidepressant medications. Because of their faster action, medications may be preferred in severe depression.

A video of his full lecture is available on You Tube (see link below.[18]

I came across an excellent article about antidepressants from Harvard Medical School that I'd like to share. It discusses how they work, how long they should be taken, why they can cause withdrawal symptoms, and what to do when you decide (in discussion with your doctor) that it's time to stop taking them.

Doctors will sometimes recommend continuing antidepressants for years to prevent depression in those who have had multiple severe bouts. But 6 months of treatment is often considered long enough treatment for a first episode. Side effects, like drowsiness, insomnia, headache, or sexual dysfunction, that are tolerable when seeking relief from depression may become bothersome and unacceptable once a person is feeling better.

Withdrawal effects that sometimes develop when discontinuing antidepressant medications can easily be confused with a return of depression itself. Working closely with a doctor while gradually decreasing the dose of the antidepressant is important. A doctor will monitor to ensure any new symptoms are caused by withdrawal and not a return of depression. A gradual taper of the medication will often be prescribed to help to minimize any withdrawal effects. When necessary, a return to a previous, slightly higher dose will ease symptoms before gradually decreasing again.

As a compounding pharmacist, I have made capsules of strengths between those commercially available to allow a more gradual dose decrease in sensitive individuals. But often withdrawal can be managed by using tablets that can be cut, liquids that can be measured in varying amounts, or by switching to longer acting medications that are cleared from the body more slowly.

If you, or someone you know, are considering stopping a long-term antidepressant medication, I'd encourage you to read more about going off antidepressants (see link below).[19]

And be sure to work closely with your doctor and your pharmacist to ensure this change is accomplished safely and as comfortably as possible.

# Antidepressants or Natural Therapies - Which works better?

The surprise answer is that most times they are equally effective.

Antidepressants have been used for decades and billions of dollars have been spent on these drugs, but their success rates are much lower than those for other types of medications, such as antibiotics for infection. The difference between the antidepressant drug effect and a placebo (or sugar pill) is almost undetectable except in more severe cases of depression. Placebos themselves are surprisingly effective, especially in less severe depression. When a person expects to get better, sometimes that is all that's needed to help the mind heal itself.

The US Centers for Disease Control and Prevention report that the rate of suicide has increased by 30% since 1999. At the same time, the use of antidepressants has increased by 65%. This suggests that, overall, the drugs are not always successful at preventing suicide, although they can be helpful in individual cases. In addition, some of these drugs have a "black box" warning, the highest level warning that can be added to a drug. It warns doctors to monitor patients for new suicidal thoughts that may occur shortly after beginning therapy.

US statistics show that greater numbers of people are on long-term financial assistance because of mental illness than before these drugs were introduced in the 1950s. One statistical analysis suggests that the drugs may actually block a full recovery, even though symptoms appear to improve in the short term. This study found that more patients who used non-drug therapies had recovered and returned to work after one to two years of treatment compared to those who took medications.

At an educational session I attended many years ago, the speaker told us that mental illnesses resulted from a chemical imbalance in the brain. Depression was caused by too little serotonin or norepinephrine. They explained that antidepressants rebalanced these chemicals (called neurotransmitters), by increasing the available levels of the ones believed to be low in depression. I often explained this to patients when I counselled them about their medication in my pharmacy.

However, newer studies have shown that the brain changes how it functions to accommodate for the effect of the drug. When the patient tries to stop the medication, it takes a while for the brain to return to normal. This manifests as symptoms of a return of the mental illness, sometimes more severe than it seemed to be before. This has often been interpreted as a need to continue treatment, rather than a withdrawal effect of the medication and can result in patients being kept on treatment for many years.

The longer the person has been taking the medication, the longer it can take for brain function to return to normal afterward. This can prolong the withdrawal time and make it very difficult to stop an antidepressant medication that has been taken for a long time. This is the reason doctors recommend tapering the dose gradually when attempting to discontinue treatment.

As well, antidepressants have side effects that range from weight gain to erectile dysfunction. The small benefit these drugs provide compared to placebo, especially in milder forms of depression, needs to be weighed against the side effects they cause. In severe depression, medication along with non-drug treatments may be necessary.

So, do studies show that alternative "natural therapies" work for depression?

The answer is yes. Good quality scientific studies are available to support some of these non-drug treatments:

1. **Exercise**
    a. A 2007 study at Duke University Medical Center in North Carolina found that 30 minutes of walking or jogging three times a week was more effective than an antidepressant or

placebo. (Psychosomatic Medicine, Sept 2007, 69(7), p. 587-96)[20]

b. A review (or "meta-analysis") of studies that included exercise and antidepressant medications in 2016 confirmed the effectiveness of exercise. (Journal of Affective Disorders, 15 Sept 2016, vol.202, p.67-86)[21]

2. **Bright light therapy**

   a. Bright light (10,000 Lux, 30-60 minutes daily first thing in the morning) attempts to duplicate the effect of being in sunshine. A review of studies[22] showed significant effect, with the largest study[23] showing an effect approximately equal to antidepressants when added to medication. Of course, spending time in actual sunshine could be expected to give the same beneficial effect.

3. **Mediterranean diet**

   a. While less studied, a small Australian study, the "SMILES Trial"[24] suggests adding a Mediterranean Diet that includes local unprocessed foods may make a greater difference than antidepressants. After 12 weeks on the diet, 32% experienced remission compared to only 8% of those who received only social support along with their other treatment. More study is needed in this area. However, eating whole local foods and mostly plants is a healthy way of eating for anyone.

4. **Cognitive behavioural therapy (CBT)**

   a. Cognitive Behaviour Therapy, or CBT, is a non-drug, "talk" therapy used to treat psychological illness. It aims to help people understand their thoughts and feelings, and what makes them feel positive, anxious or depressed. It helps people to identify the problems that are troubling them and find different ways to think and behave to manage their feelings.

   b. The evidence for benefit from CBT is indisputable.[25] It is

> as effective as antidepressants but, unlike medication, the
> effect continues after the therapy is completed. The other
> plus is that a person can't overdose on a bottle of "therapy",
> unlike antidepressants...

So, if you get the "blues" next winter, talk to your doctor. But, before they take out the prescription pad, be sure to ask whether non-drug therapies might be appropriate for you. While you may benefit from medication, or a combination of medication and non-drug therapy, it's worthwhile discussing your options first.

Of course, considering the positive effect of exercise, sunshine, a healthy diet and discussing ways to deal with problems effectively with someone you trust, perhaps these are things we should all be doing every day anyway to keep our bodies and our minds healthy!

References:

Anatomy of an Epidemic, by Robert Whittaker

Why Natural Depression Therapies are Better Than Pills, Dr. Matt Strauss (Pharmacy Practice Journal) http://www.canadianhealthcarenetwork.ca/pharmacists/discussions/why-natural-depression-therapies-are-better-than-pills-43441?utm_source=EmailMark

# Chapter 12: The Last Word...

Much of this book originated as part of a series of weekly blogs. One reason I blog each week is to investigate new ideas and learn more about being healthy myself, both mentally and physically, while I find ideas to share and answer questions from readers. Satisfying my curiosity, I suppose, and yours at the same time...

If you enjoyed the ideas in this book, I'm sure you would like my weekly blog. You can sign up for free at http://jeanniebeaudin.wixsite.com/Author to have a link delivered directly to your inbox each week, usually on Friday.

Hope to see you there!

Jeannie

---

[1] http://jeanniebeaudin.wixsite.com/author/single-post/2018/12/[1]07/Antidepressants-or-Natural-Therapies—-Which-works-better[2]

[2] https://movingmedicine.ac.uk/

[3] https://www.ncbi.nlm.nih.gov/pubmed/29044440

[4] https://www.who.int/news-room/fact-sheets/detail/physical-activity

[5] http://www.tobaccoinaustralia.org.au/chapter-1-prevalence/1-13[3]-international-comparisons-of-prevalence-of-sm[4]

---

1. http://jeanniebeaudin.wixsite.com/author/single-post/2018/12/07/
   Antidepressants-or-Natural-Therapies---Which-works-better

2. http://jeanniebeaudin.wixsite.com/author/single-post/2018/12/07/
   Antidepressants-or-Natural-Therapies---Which-works-better

3. http://www.tobaccoinaustralia.org.au/chapter-1-prevalence/
   1-13-international-comparisons-of-prevalence-of-sm

4. http://www.tobaccoinaustralia.org.au/chapter-1-prevalence/
   1-13-international-comparisons-of-prevalence-of-sm

[6]Deprescribing information for PPI's http://cfp.ca/content/63/5/354.full

[7] http://www.karger.com/Article/PDF/381654

[8] http://www.ravnskov.nu/cm/

[9] https://www.nhlbi.nih.gov/health-topics/dash-eating-plan

[10] https://www.townhallmedicine.com/summit-themes/

[11]      http://jeanniebeaudin.wixsite.com/author/single-post/2016/07/[5]22/
Bacteria-for-Breakfast-Probiotics-for-Good-Health-%E2%80%93
[6]-A-book-review[7]

[12]                  http://www.mayoclinic.org/diseases-conditions/obesity/
in-depth[8]/bmi-calculator/itt-20084938[9]

[13] http://onlinelibrary.wiley.com/doi/10.1038/oby.2009.191/full

[14] https://www.plasticpollutioncoalition.org/.

[15] http://www.mybraintrainer.com/

[16] https://mysleepwell.ca/

[17]                        https://www.nytimes.com/2018/08/14/style/
how-can-i-focus-better.html?rref=collection%2Fsectioncollection%2Fsmarter-livin

---


5. http://jeanniebeaudin.wixsite.com/author/single-post/2016/07/22/
   Bacteria-for-Breakfast-Probiotics-for-Good-Health-%E2%80%93-A-book-review

6. http://jeanniebeaudin.wixsite.com/author/single-post/2016/07/22/
   Bacteria-for-Breakfast-Probiotics-for-Good-Health-%E2%80%93-A-book-review

7. http://jeanniebeaudin.wixsite.com/author/single-post/2016/07/22/
   Bacteria-for-Breakfast-Probiotics-for-Good-Health-%E2%80%93-A-book-review

8. http://www.mayoclinic.org/diseases-conditions/obesity/in-depth/bmi-calculator/itt-20084938

9. http://www.mayoclinic.org/diseases-conditions/obesity/in-depth/bmi-calculator/itt-20084938

[18] https://www.youtube.com/watch?v=NOAgplgTxfc

[19] https://www.health.harvard.edu/diseases-and-conditions/going-off-antidepressants

[20] https://www.researchgate.net/publication/5994774_Exercise_and_Pharmacotherapy_in_the_Treatment_of_Major_Depressive

[21] https://www.sciencedirect.com/science/article/pii/S0165032715314221?via%3Dihub

[22] https://www.sciencedirect.com/science/article/pii/S0165032716300076?via%3Dihub

[23] https://onlinelibrary.wiley.com/doi/abs/10.1111/j.1600-0447.2005.00574.x

[24] https://bmcmedicine.biomedcentral.com/articles/10.1186/s12916-017-0791-y

[25] https://journals.sagepub.com/doi/10.1177/070674371305800702

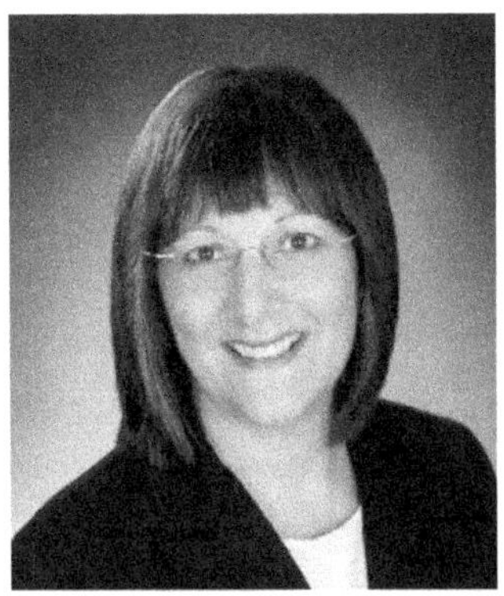

# About the Author

Jeannie Collins Beaudin is a recently retired pharmacist with 40 years experience in community pharmacy and specialty compounding. She has also been a columnist and blogger for a national pharmacy journal, Pharmacy Practice + Business, since 2006.

In her personal blog, http://jeanniebeaudin.wixsite.com/author, she shares health information, news, opinions, ideas and controversies based on scientific research and her experience as a community compounding pharmacist and hormone specialist.

Jeannie has given many presentations over the years to highly varied groups, from information sessions at her store, to office lunch-and-learns, to professional groups at conferences... on varied topics from hormones, natural medicine and compounding pharmacy to cancer prevention and seniors' health. Audiences have included the general public, health professionals, students and a few web conferences (webinars!).

You can contact Jeannie through her website (above) or at Jeannie.Beaudin@gmail.com .

Read more at jeanniebeaudin.wixsite.com/author.